Nurse-facilitated discharge from hospital

Forthcoming titles from M&K Publishing

Improving Patient Outcomes: A Guide for Ward Managers
ISBN 978-1-905539-06-1

Modern Management in Chronic Disease and Long-Term Conditions
ISBN 978-1-905539-15-4

The ECG Workbook
ISBN 978-1-905539-14-7

The Advanced Respiratory Practitioner:
A Practical and Theoretical Guide for Nurses and AHPs
ISBN 978-1-905539-10-9

Pre-Operative Assessment and Perioperative Management
ISBN 978-1-905539-02-9

Pre-Teen and Teenage Pregnancy: A 21st-Century Reality
ISBN 978-1-905539-11-8

Eye Emergencies: The Practitioner's Guide
ISBN 978-1-905539-08-6

Managing Emotions in Women's Health
ISBN 978-1-905539-07-X

Ionising Radiation (Medical Exposure) Regulations
– Theory Training Module
ISBN 978-1-905539-04-8

Ward-based Critically Ill Patients: A Guide for Health Professionals
ISBN 978-1-905539-03-1

The Management of Pain in Older People
ISBN 978-1-905539-22-2

Prescribing for Advanced Medical Practitioners
Working in Musculoskeletal Medicine
ISBN 978-1-905539-09-3

Nurse-facilitated discharge from hospital

Edited by

Liz Lees
Consultant Nurse (Acute Medicine),
Birmingham Heart of England NHS Foundation Trust.

M&K Publishing
©2006 M&K Update Ltd

First published 2007

Notice:
Clinical practice and medical knowledge constantly evolve. Standard safety precautions must be followed, but as knowledge is broadened by research, changes in practice, treatment and drug therapy may become necessary or appropriate. Readers must check the most current product information provided by the manufacturer of each drug to be administered and verify the dosages and correct administration, as well as contraindications. It is the responsibility of the practitioner, utilising the experience and knowledge of the patient, to determine dosages and the best treatment for each individual patient. Neither the publisher nor the authors assume any liability for any injury and/or damage to persons or property arising from this publication.

The Publisher

To contact M&K Publishing write to:
M&K Update Ltd · The Old Bakery · St John's Street · Keswick · Cumbria · CA12 5AS
a part of M&K Update Ltd

Tel: 01768 773030 · Fax: 01768 781099
publishing@mkupdate.co.uk
www.mkupdate.co.uk

British Library Cataloguing in Publication Data
A catalogue record for this book is available from the British Library

ISBN: 978-1-905539-12-3

Designed and illustrated by Mary Blood
Typeset in 11pt Usherwood Book
Printed in the United Kingdom by Reed's Limited

Acknowledgements

To my colleagues:
I have always had a lot to say, but thanks to you all I have been able to say even more, thank you.

To FIona Macdonald:
I could not have compiled and edited this book without your superb patience and support.

To my employers:
Birmingham Heart of England NHS Foundation Trust. Thank you for being the test bed for new and innovative discharge practice.

Contents

List of contributors

Ros Moore (Foreword)
Professional Officer for Acute Nursing,
Department of Health, Quarry House, Quarry Hill, Leeds

Liz Lees (Preface, Chapters 1 and 16)
Consultant Nurse (Acute Medicine),
Birmingham Heart of England NHS Foundation Trust
and
Visiting Lecturer, University of Central England, Birmingham

Tracey Riley (Chapter 2)
Director of Medical Events,
M&K Update Ltd, Cumbria

Ann Saxon (Chapter 3)
Principal Lecturer for Post-graduate Studies,
School of Health, University of Wolverhampton

Denise Price (Chapter 4)
Assistant Director of Nursing,
Education and Workforce Planning
Birmingham Heart of England NHS Foundation Trust

Lyn Garbarino (Chapter 4)
Head of Workforce Development and Training,
North Cumbria Mental Health and Learning Disabilities NHS Trust

Alison Wells (Chapter 5)
Independent consultant,
Professionally based in Leicester

Dr Philip Dyer (Chapter 6)
Consultant Physician (Acute Medicine),
Diabetes and Endocrinology
and
Lead Consultant (Emergency Assessment Area),
Birmingham Heart of England NHS Foundation Trust

Dr Mark Temple (Chapter 6)
Associate Medical Director (Emergency Care)
Birmingham Heart of England NHS Foundation Trust

Siân Wade (Chapters 7 and 15)
Multi-professional Clinical Educator (Elderly Care Directorate),
Birmingham Heart of England NHS Foundation Trust

Lorraine Marsh (Chapter 8)
Senior Occupational Therapist,
Birmingham Heart of England NHS Foundation Trust

Contributors

Jo Brady (Chapter 8)
Occupational Therapist,
Birmingham Heart of England NHS Foundation Trust

Ross Groves (Chapter 9)
Independent pharmacy consultant

Lynn Beun (Chapter 10)
Service Improvement Facilitator,
Brighton and Sussex University Hospitals NHS Trust

Bob McMaster (Chapter 11)
Consultant Nurse (Emergency Departments)
Leeds Teaching Hospitals NHS Trust

Karen Tongue (Chapter 12)
Matron (ENT/Ophthalmology)
Birmingham Heart of England NHS Foundation Trust

Andrea Field (Chapter 13)
Matron (Acute Medicine)
Birmingham Heart of England NHS Foundation Trust

Ann Edgar (Chapter 14)
Matron for Rehabilitation (Elderly Care Directorate)
Birmingham Heart of England NHS Foundation Trust

Barbara Mason (Chapter 16)
Advanced Nurse Practitioner
Birmingham East and North Primary Care Trust

Foreword

I was delighted to be asked to write the foreword for a book that addresses what is still one of the most important but variable aspects of patient experience, but one where nurses can really make a difference.

Improving hospital discharge remains at the centre of the government's drive to improve standards and cut waiting times. A great deal has been achieved already and the Healthcare Commission in-patient survey published in May 2006 showed sustained improvements. However, 38 per cent of the patients surveyed still experienced delayed discharge because they were waiting for medication or a doctor. The quality of information provided when leaving hospital was also still a problem. More than 40 per cent said they were discharged without being told about the side-effects of medication. And 40 per cent said that they were not told about the danger signals they should watch out for once they were at home. Almost 25 per cent were not told what to do if they were worried about their condition after leaving hospital (www.healthcarecommission.org.uk).

Getting discharge right benefits everyone: patients feel better and the hospital is able to employ its valuable resources to maximum effect. Failures on the other hand are potentially costly, undermining staff morale and public confidence and leading to poor patient outcomes.

The potential for nurses to improve patient discharge has long been recognised. In 2004, the Department of Health, picking up on the Chief Nursing Officer's 'Ten key roles for nurses' (2000), published 'Achieving a timely 'simple' discharge from hospital'. This document recommended that senior nurses should be empowered to facilitate the discharge of patients.

As we can see from this book, nurses have been rising to this challenge – while breaking down many of the structural and cultural barriers that have inhibited progress in the past. However, the Healthcare Commission survey serves as a timely reminder that there is still some way to go.

As time goes on, discharge will increasingly take place in a patient-led system, where more choice of provider will lead to

Foreword

greater quality and productivity. More care will be provided in the home and community, and patient choice and global mobility will result in patients being treated away from home or abroad.

In this context, discharge will be focused on the needs and concerns of patients, not on the needs of clinicians or the service as a whole. The drive towards integrated healthcare and social care will demand a seamless service, capable of working across geographical and cultural boundaries.

This book on nurse-facilitated discharge therefore comes at exactly the right time. Facilitation clearly places the nurse as coordinator and facilitative leader of discharge, rather than its director. It emphasises the real partnership between patients, carers and professions that must lie at the centre of discharge, especially for the growing number of older people living with long-term conditions. Nurse-facilitated discharge will be characterised by proactive, personalised, holistic planning; multidisciplinary and inter-agency team working; good communications, efficient processes and the innovative use of information and assistive technology. It will see the nurse acting as coordinator, technician, clinical expert, teacher, resource person, advocate and counsellor.

This book is a good reference resource for those wishing to move in this direction and improve hospital discharge for patients today and in the future.

Ros Moore
Professional Officer for Acute Nursing
Department of Health
July 2006

Preface

This book discusses nurse-facilitated discharge in the context of an acute hospital setting. However, nurses facilitate the process of discharge and the transfer of patients in many other healthcare settings, and the principles of practice illustrated are easily transferable. This book is presented in three distinct sections: background and theory, clinical practice considerations and case studies. This approach, including both the theoretical and practical aspects of hospital discharge, should make the book a valuable reference tool in practice settings.

Section 1 ('Background and theory') starts with Chapter 1, which explores a broad range of issues affecting hospital discharge. In particular, it looks at government policy and some of the core issues, such as change management, bed management and team working. A distinction is also drawn between nurse-led and nurse-facilitated discharge from hospital. And, it discusses leadership, responsibility and accountability in relation to expanding the nursing role in discharge planning. Chapter 2 addresses some of the core theoretical and organisational issues that need to be taken into account when developing a hospital discharge policy. Chapter 3 covers educational frameworks and collaboration between university providers to deliver new courses on hospital discharge. Finally, Chapter 4 outlines the knowledge skills framework and the development of competency that together pave the way for nurse-facilitated discharge.

Section 2 ('Clinical practice considerations') begins with Chapter 5, which outlines the action needed at board level to achieve strategic momentum within an organisation. Without the support of practice development departments, the discharge planning process can easily fragment into pockets of good practice or not be adopted at all. Medical support for nurse-facilitated discharge is a subject that is rarely addressed in any detail, yet it can play a crucial role. Chapter 6 explores the key issues in detail, particularly the decision-making process, the function of ward rounds, shared learning opportunities and the development of robust management plans. Chapter 7 discusses the role of nurses, emphasising their multidisciplinary function when dealing with complex issues to effect a good quality of discharge. It consolidates

Preface

many points made throughout previous chapters but addresses patient outcomes supported by case examples from practice. Chapter 8 offers a definition of occupational therapy and explains the occupational therapist's role in relation to discharge planning. This chapter should assist understanding of the many interfaces between occupational therapists and nursing and the approaches used in assessment for discharge. Finally, Chapter 9 discusses discharge medication. Organisations often tackle the engagement of pharmacists in the discharge process from a purely management perspective. Here, patient assessment on admission, the pharmacist's role, nurse prescribing and many other approaches to prescribing discharge medication are discussed in relation to patient outcomes.

Section 3 ('Case studies') includes seven case studies written by practitioners working in a variety of settings. Throughout this section, aspects covered in other chapters will be consolidated and new light will be shed on theoretical issues discussed earlier. This section should therefore set a clear direction for those practitioners wishing to introduce new ways of safely discharging patients.

Liz Lees
September 2006

Section 1

Background and theory

Chapter 1

Exploring nurse-facilitated discharge from hospital

Liz Lees

The core elements in good discharge planning are:
- Clear policy on hospital discharge
- Effective change management processes
- Ward coordination: role and functions
- Leadership skills
- Good skills in patient assessment
- Competency development
- Discharge training

Policy on hospital discharge

Policy on discharge

Many of the principles underpinning discharge planning remain the same as they have always been, despite the enormous changes that have taken place in the National Health Service since its inception. Perhaps the biggest challenges in discharge planning today arise from shorter lengths of patient stay, increasing patient throughput, and the acuteness of a patient's medical condition when they are admitted to hospital. The gradual and sustained development of new roles for nurses, combined with medical advances, has also played a large part. Changes in the NHS have led to altered patient/carer needs and expectations. This has required the commissioning of new patient-ßcentred services, which have in turn stimulated further changes in discharge planning practice (DoH 2002a, 2005a, b). Policy documents have reflected these changes by placing more emphasis on specific areas of discharge practice and, in particular, on nurses' contribution to these areas (DoH 2003a).

Background and theory

In most cases, new policy leads to new ways of working. In others, it may provide additional support for a change already being practised by nurses. In the case of discharge planning, policy appears to have reawakened interest in the nurse's role. This happened most noticeably after the announcement of the Chief Nursing Officer's 'Ten key roles for nurses' (DoH 2000). The 'admitting and discharging patients' key role elevated discharge practice from an arguably routine task to a high-profile function to be incorporated in different ways into nurses' delivery of patient care. Nevertheless, achieving practical success in this key role depends upon many different organisational facets working together. It also has an impact upon numerous professional groups within the NHS, requiring them to adjust their roles in discharge planning.

Single assessment process

The Single Assessment Process was introduced shortly after the 'National Service Framework for Older People' was published (DoH 2001a, b). Much of the work involved in implementing this framework rested with nurses. While the process of implementation was initially arduous, its intention was to simplify and integrate assessments. It also provided a basis for healthcare and social care professionals to work together in new ways. For example, both groups were encouraged to get involved at the outset in patient assessment, and then carry out thorough discharge planning for patients. This required nurses to step outside their traditional role in hospitals, to integrate professional practices and organisational systems, in order to guide the patient's discharge (DoH 2002b). However, in many cases the abundance of policy is not necessarily supported by the organisational changes required to implement it. This continues to be a challenge in many practice settings today.

A noteworthy, inspiring guidance document entitled 'The Freedom to Practise' illustrated emergency care policy in practice settings by providing case examples of patient care from the point of referral to the point of discharge. Encouragingly, this included mechanisms to facilitate nurse leadership in the discharge process (RCN & DoH 2003). This radical policy document gave nurses tangible support in taking on a leadership role in discharging patients within everyday clinical practice.

A second area of policy focus, reiterated in several documents, recommended naming key individuals to act as discharge coordinators at ward level (modules 4a and 4b of www.dischargetraining .doh.gov.uk). Some may argue that this is not a new concept at all and probably has its roots in systems of ward organisation, leadership at the ward level and management (Martin 2006). Whatever its origins, having a named discharge coordinator provided members of the multidisciplinary team (including doctors) and other agencies with a specific person to liaise with when coordinating the discharge plan (DoH 2003b). This policy indicated pathway, process and plan. Furthermore, it included a specific renewed emphasis on discharge checklists as part of the process (Lees 2006a).

This policy guidance was virtually a directive and was reinforced at hospital Board level through its inclusion as a measurable facet of Trust performance in the Clinical Negligence Scheme for Trusts (DoH 2003c). The CNST stipulates that there should be a named person in the discharge plan, and that there should be a checklist. These two elements provide a quantifiable audit trail in order to determine that the various stages in the discharge process have taken place (Lees 2006a).

At the same time, changes in the funding of patients delayed in hospital (while they wait for social care provision to be put in place) brought about another process known as recharging (DoH, LAC 21: 2003d). Recharging is inextricably linked with discharge, and therefore requires nurses to instigate it. However, recharging can also be seen as a separate or even parallel task. Recharging has a major impact on the process of estimating dates of medical fitness to discharge and that of estimating the length of stay or discharge date itself (see Chapter 6).

Finally, talk of timely discharge to stimulate simple discharges from hospital saw the introduction of another toolkit 'Achieving timely 'simple' discharge from hospital' (DoH 2004a). In this policy document, the nurse's role was reasserted and embraced. Yet national evidence reveals highly disparate practice, ranging from well-developed innovative local policy and protocols to small-scale projects with little strategic support to sustain them (see Section 3, 'Case studies').

The sustainable introduction of innovative discharge practice depends overwhelmingly on the nursing profession, supported by members of the multidisciplinary team. And the discharge process is vitally important, even though many nurses may perceive it as being dominated by paperwork and systems of collecting data. Nonetheless, to achieve the magnitude of change required, directors, service/operational managers and other allied healthcare practitioners must also be prepared to examine their working practices for the benefit of patients and join in with the process of change. Organisational readiness is imperative in order to support nurses. Nursing professionals cannot achieve the scale of change required on their own. Their links with other practitioners are vital in balancing policy, and in understanding and implementing the concept of nurse-facilitated hospital discharge.

Change management processes

'Ten key roles for nurses' (DoH 2000b) created new opportunities for some nurses and increased responsibilities for others, depending on the extent to which they were already proactively involved in changing the planning and implementation of hospital discharge. The changes required will stimulate the development of new organisational policies, protocols and training, which will assist both the employing organisation and the individual practitioner in expanding their role and taking on new practices (Lees & Emmerson 2006). It will also promote the development of new teams and instigate innovative ways of working to benefit the patient. Finally, the scale of change will elicit integrated working practices outside hospital, involving the many different organisations that deliver healthcare and social care.

Despite this positive perspective, change can be quite a frightening prospect for some professionals, and it has not always been readily adopted in the area of discharge practice. For example, while researching this book it has become evident that protective mechanisms are sometimes adopted by individual professionals to preserve the status quo in their particular profession. This tendency is often reinforced by oppressive strategies used to deliberately slow down the pace of change, especially if it is believed that the change will have an adverse impact on role development (Leason 2003).

To counterbalance possible misapprehensions and resulting tensions, organisations should aim to develop a culture of sustaining new practices in the long term. A short-term approach is only likely to impede development or shorten the shelf-life of the change. Therefore, change must be managed effectively, and preparation, planning and discussion are crucial to ensure success. This is particularly important when change is occurring because of wider agendas and priorities that may not be apparent to those working at practice level.

Bed management

Bed management

Bed management is not a new concept; indeed it is a fundamental aspect of every hospital's 24-hour working day (National Audit Office 2003). So why is it often seen as separate from nursing? Bed management started as part of nursing, but it has migrated to become a separate aspect of management. This separation of roles makes it more difficult for nurses to proactively manage the processes of patient admission and discharge.

There are many texts that explore capacity management and large organisational systems. Yet, perhaps partly because of their distance from the practice mindset of most nurses, they tend to be regarded with little interest by nurses. It could be argued that lack of bed capacity, and intensive turnover of patients with a higher acuteness of medical condition, creates untoward pressure. This in itself counteracts the notion of 'caring for patients' and promotes a culture of 'counting patient throughput'. Bed management posts were originally created to relieve pressure on nurses, yet this role most certainly requires nursing input. Asking the following questions may reveal a constructive way forward:

- What do we want those responsible for bed management to achieve?
- What approach to bed management should they use?
- Is a universal role the answer?

At present, a variety of bed management models can be seen throughout the UK. These include: not having any defined system or bed manager, corporate administrative teams, clinical bed coordinators, incorporating the bed management function as part of an operational manager's role, strategic bed managers, and computerised data entry systems (only as reliable as the person entering the data!).

Ideally, the nurse's unique knowledge of the patient should be combined with knowledge of bed management systems and processes, adopting a 'can do' or problem-solving approach. At the Heart of England Foundation Trust in Birmingham a non clinical corporate bed management team is supported by clinically based bed co-ordinators, who are responsible for practice in their own clinical area. This system allocates responsibility for the discharge. It also enables clinical coordination of the patient's needs in order to free the hospital bed earlier in the day.

The system is not without its own problems. First, all areas of practice need to adopt the same approach in order to achieve the same momentum across the organisation, especially when patients need to transfer within the hospital rather than being discharged. Secondly, cost effectiveness needs to be assessed, alongside freed bed capacity, patients' satisfaction and patient-centred care. If these factors are not taken into account, clinical bed coordinators may be regarded as an expensive luxury – once again 'here today and gone tomorrow'. This said, bed management and proactive systems to free up beds earlier in the day are constantly evolving.

Team working

Team working

Team working could be argued to be in a state of demise, with the nurse's role largely centred on coordinating a 'group' as opposed to a 'team' of staff working together on a shift (Martin 2006). Understanding the difference between a 'group' and a 'team' may provide some valuable clues as to where some discharge planning problems originate. For example, a ward team can be defined as a team made up of consistent staff members, with clearly defined roles (Belbin 1993), belonging to that ward or clinical area. In addition, a team will have a shared or common purpose (Martin 2006), such as achieving the discharge plan within a defined timescale. This is hugely important in terms of representing the patient's perspective along what may be quite a complex route to discharge from hospital (Tierney 2000).

Perhaps the systems that have been established to manage services are part of the problem? For instance, staff members are frequently moved between wards to ensure safe staffing levels. Agency and bank nurses, while crucially needed, are often used to 'top up levels of staff' to established levels per shift. Moreover, temporary wards are often opened at times of additional pressure (summer and winter included), to increase the bed capacity on a flexible basis, using staff available at short notice and agency or bank nurses, who may not know each other's strengths or specialist skills.

Furthermore, such temporary wards are often closed at short notice. This has a catastrophic effect on the essential communication and handover involved in discharge, such as putting together a patient discharge plan (which is a multi-professional and coordinated activity, though one that is usually facilitated by nurses). Organisational practices of this nature will lead to fragmented communication, limiting the development of nurses' knowledge and extending patient lengths of stay. They are also likely to lead to a lack of ownership of discharge planning (Pethybridge 2004).

A team includes allied health professionals and doctors as well as nurses, and a team should accept responsibility and grow in knowledge and skills (Martin 2006). It could be argued that changes such as reducing junior doctors' working hours and moving away from ward-based teams of doctors have had a negative effect on our concept of a team. These changes have also shifted more responsibility on to nurses, who have the greatest patient contact, spread over 24 hours a day, 7 days a week. Perhaps nurses are in a position to assert some control by stating what they need (tools and resources) and how they need to work (Kuockkanen & Kilpi 2000). Without doubt, achieving effective nurse-facilitated hospital discharge will require strong leadership from nursing.

Leadership skills

Leadership skills

'Passion, drive and commitment' are three essential aspects of developing a culture of nurse leadership, irrespective of the particular subject being explored (Martin 2006). When it comes to discharge planning, passion may arise from knowledge of the subject and the desire to carry out the role. In addition, understanding the organisational goals will give nurses a sense of ownership and a desire to be proactively involved in patient discharge.

Drive and commitment go hand in hand, particularly in discharge planning, where it is crucial to track the progress of a problem until it is resolved. For example, rather than 'leaving an issue to chance', by handing it over to others or disowning it altogether, it should be followed through, regardless of shift pattern or which professional it was handed to. Differing acuteness of patients' medical conditions and frequent complexity of care make it notoriously difficult to keep track of who did what, what the result was, and what its implications were for patient care. All this will impact on the discharge plan and possibly on the patient's length of stay (see 'Case example 1' below). It therefore requires a significant commitment from the nurse to take responsibility and focus upon creating a discharge plan, as a priority, along with the many other aspects of nursing care that require delivery. Leading the plan requires sustained commitment to regularly review the patient's progress and to assert control.

Case example 1

Case example 1

Junior doctors on an acute medical ward made a physiotherapy referral for an oxygen saturation assessment and mobility assessment, only to discover that the physiotherapist had already discharged the patient from her care earlier in the week. In this case, the central factors in the discharge plan were not stated at the outset of care. While individual therapy referrals had been made, the patient was effectively waiting in a queue for a series of single unconnected events to take place. This left the desired outcome uncertain and open-ended.

Achieving a leadership mentality requires nurses to question the way they organise themselves to deliver care. Nurses often say that they feel overwhelmed by activities and tasks, but organisation and leadership help to create valuable time. For example, in the case of discharge planning and the busy acute hospital environment, nurses may get too tied up in individual tasks, rather than understanding where they are in the process and thereby which tasks will achieve the biggest impact in the time they have. There is an overwhelming need to clarify the patient's individual needs with all the professionals involved, over an approximate indicated timescale, in a discharge plan (Lees *et al.* 2006a, Lees & Holmes 2005, Kuockkanen & Kilpi 2000). This discussion must be based on the principles, the process and the desired outcome (see 'Fundamental principles of discharge planning' below).

Principles of discharge planning

Fundamental principles of discharge planning

1. Knowledge of disease process or condition
2. **Estimating how long recovery might take, or if recovery is a realistic outcome**
3. **Involving the patient and family and carers in the plan**
4. Proactively dealing with issues and difficulties that may arise
5. Communicating and documenting the plan to the team or group of staff
6. Making appropriate referrals and following through outcomes
7. Coordinating and owning the discharge information
8. Being decisive and carrying out activities
9. **Reviewing and updating the progress of the plan**
10. Disseminating accurate information to all involved

Evidence from the case notes of patients who have had reasonably short lengths of stay (perhaps less than three days) indicates that three of these principles (2, 3 and 9) are quite commonly overlooked. If these three aspects were routinely addressed, nurses could assert a greater degree of control and ownership of the discharge process and this would benefit patient care. In addition, leadership provided by nurse executives/directors should be actively utilised by experienced nurses to develop the appropriate infrastructure and to guide the processes required. All these actions will promote the principle of working in partnership with the patient, the patient's family and the multidisciplinary team towards effective nurse-facilitated discharge practice (DoH 2004).

Nurse-led or nurse-facilitated hospital discharge?

Nursing literature has focused a great deal of attention upon the term used to discuss the role of nurses in relation to the discharge process (Rudd & Smith 2002, Lees 2004). According to some consultants and other healthcare practitioners, the name adopted is incredibly important. For example, the term 'nurse-led' implies a uni-disciplinary activity. This idea can generate bad feeling and fear that patients will be discharged without appropriate management from medical and allied health professional colleagues. In the nursing field, it can also have undesirable effects, such as causing hospital discharge to be seen as a role exclusively reserved for only a privileged, adequately prepared/trained minority. Debating the appropriate terminology may be time consuming, but it can serve a useful purpose by making the intended goals explicit. Moreover, in determining organisational discharge policy, this discussion can pave the way for the implementation of new and innovative practices.

Definition of terms

The term **'nurse-facilitated'** is derived from a set of behaviours required to complete the discharge process (see 'Fundamental principles of discharge planning', p.11). For example, nurse-facilitated discharge can be defined as 'a process where nurses take responsibility for the proactive management of discharge of patients in their care from hospital'.

The term **'nurse-led'** has been defined as 'nurses leading the whole process of discharge, following decisions made by nurses, using criteria, protocols or a given set of principles' (adapted from Lees 2006b).

Regardless of which name is adopted, discharge should never be seen as the sole responsibility of senior nurses, nurse specialists or nurse consultants. Nor should it be conducted in isolation, without the support of all appropriate members of the multidisciplinary team.

Some of the fears expressed by other healthcare practitioners can perhaps be allayed by formulating a list of undesirable and desirable actions for nurses involved in the discharge process.

Nurses facilitating discharge should *not*:

- Carry out a series of instructions as indicated by the medical team. (When it comes to discharge, nurses should be the facilitators.)
- Decide a patient is fit for discharge without consulting the relevant professionals involved with the patient's care.
- Wait for the doctor to make decisions about discharge when the nurse has had the relevant training/knowledge to make those decisions.

- Discharge a patient according to different rules depending who is in charge of the ward and/or on duty.
- Discharge patients without preparing them adequately, when there are bed capacity issues.

Nurses facilitating discharge *should*:

- Initiate and lead the discharge process with involvement of all relevant professionals to expedite discharges, and assist bed and capacity management across the whole hospital.
- Carry out regular and ongoing patient assessments/evaluations to assist timely and appropriate discharges.
- Progress-chase the results of investigations that require the nurse's decision to expedite discharge.
- Proactively engage the multidisciplinary team at appropriate points in the patient's care.
- Proactively promote and discuss discharge decisions, in collaboration with the patient's family and the multidisciplinary team to promote discharges.
- Follow up the patient (in and out of hospital) and review progress, according to the discharge plan.
- Act as the patient's advocate.

(Adapted from Lees 2004)

It has been suggested that nurses learn new ways of behaving, and reframe their professional image, role and values. In fact, nurses facilitating patient discharge are already trying to clarify their roles and responsibilities in the multiple stages of the discharge process. This clarity will benefit both the patients and the organisation.

A few NHS organisations have made drastic changes in their nurse-facilitated discharge practices, transferring the main burden of responsibility for patient discharge (previously shouldered by doctors and therapists) on to nurses. Some nurses regard this expansion and adjustment as a natural evolution of their role, while others argue that it amounts to carrying out a doctor's duties for a nurse's pay.

Nonetheless, nurse-facilitated discharge provides a positive step forward. The diagram below places 'nurse-facilitated' and 'nurse-led' on a continuum of development. With this in mind, nurses need to have a good understanding of their parameters of practice and be aware of their individual responsibility and accountability (NMC 2004).

Background and theory

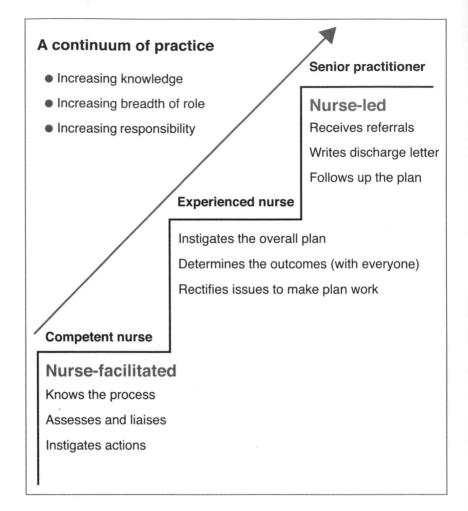

A continuum of practice

- Increasing knowledge
- Increasing breadth of role
- Increasing responsibility

Senior practitioner

Nurse-led

Receives referrals

Writes discharge letter

Follows up the plan

Experienced nurse

Instigates the overall plan

Determines the outcomes (with everyone)

Rectifies issues to make plan work

Competent nurse

Nurse-facilitated

Knows the process

Assesses and liaises

Instigates actions

Exploring responsibility and accountability

Responsibility

There is often some reluctance to embrace nurse-facilitated discharge in certain parts of an organisation. For example, attitudes and practice may differ from ward to ward. This is partly because, until relatively recently, there were few organisational policies and protocols to support nursing actions in practice. However, there are no longer any legal or professional obstacles to nurses taking increasing responsibility for the discharge process, including the decision to discharge a patient (DoH 2004). In addition, the Royal College of Nursing actively supports nurses' involvement in the process (RCN 2000). Specifically, local policy is essential to ensure that the value of nurse-facilitated discharge in practice settings is recognised at all levels of the organisation (CNST: DoH 2003c).

Responsibility

Perhaps it is the individual interpretation of 'nurse-facilitated discharge' that is self-limiting nurses in practice? Evidence suggests that many nurses fear the 'responsibility' of being left alone to contemplate a discharge decision, where perhaps not all the issues are resolved or further clarity is required. Moreover, guarded behaviour is evident when nurses believe the responsibility is not 'theirs' to take. The issue is compounded when junior and senior members of the medical teams express anxiety that their patients may be discharged without their prior knowledge or consent.

Conversely, some nurses do lead and coordinate all discharges from hospital in their area of practice, with the absolute support of their medical colleagues. Indeed, it may be considered an insult to these nurses to suggest that they have ever practised any other way. The degree of responsibility shouldered by a nurse facilitating a discharge will vary tremendously, depending on the expertise of the particular nurse. The same can be said of junior doctors, some of whom may admit patients as a safeguard, and some of whom may delay a discharge decision until their senior colleagues are present. The most important aspects of nurse-facilitated discharge to remember are that:

- Knowledge of the patient is a prerequisite
- Training is required
- Experience is essential
- Patient discharge is not a uni-disciplinary activity
- The patient must be reviewed and be medically fit for discharge

Accountability

The Nursing and Midwifery Council (NMC 2004) has stated the professional standards that provide the foundation of nursing practice. Central to these standards are nurses' decisions to act or not act, and to act in the best interests of the patient. These guiding principles can be applied to nurse-facilitated discharge from hospital. It is vital to understand what nurse facilitation involves in order to assess whether sufficient preparation for discharge has been undertaken.

Rather than being influenced by fear of negative consequences (such as possible removal from the register or litigation), nurses' decision-making should be informed by knowledge of the account-ability framework. Rudd and Smith (2002) believe that nurses should proactively take the lead in coordinating discharge planning. Nurse-facilitated discharge involves assessing the patient, liaising with the multidisciplinary team, and planning timely discharge based on the agreed plan of care (RCN & DoH 2003, DoH 2004). Writing discharge letters, making follow-up calls, and advising patients, carers and other professionals, are also within the scope of the nurse's role in discharge planning (NMC 2004, DoH 2004, RCN & DoH 2003).

Making decisions within agreed parameters requires experience and professional judgement. However, these levels of experience and judgement are not necessarily reflected by a nurse's pay banding or job title. Experience in the role through proven activities is desirable, but it should be acknowledged that some discharge issues are extremely complex and require supreme confidence to deal with effectively.

Competency development

Competency development

Chapter 4 of this book explores the competency framework developed by the Royal College of Nursing (RCN 2006) in detail. However, in view of the emphasis being placed on competency achievement in nursing as well as in other professions, it may be helpful to introduce the subject briefly here.

The development of NHS roles through prerequisite knowledge and skills is now supported by 'The NHS Knowledge and Skills Framework' (DoH 2004b). Competencies underpin this framework and provide the detail needed to encourage individual practitioners to progress through different levels of the trajectory (RCN 2006). This will in turn provide 'expanded' practice to support new services. However, competency 'development' is often misinterpreted as being task orientated. People assume that training is required to enable a series of individual tasks to be performed. These extended practices may then be hurriedly introduced, producing a superficial and constrained approach to developing the practice needs of the workforce (Bargargliotti *et al.* 1999). This is perhaps partly why the NHS has a history of short-term change projects. These short-term change projects do not necessarily interlink with established services. As a result they can end up being seen as 'stand-alone', which may have the effect of marginalising the person, role and service.

To take the first step towards creating appropriate competencies, a thorough understanding of discharge planning in context is required. This needs to include an understanding of the ward team, the services the patient is being discharged from and to, and other interfacing roles/services (Bharr 1998).

It is perfectly possible that all the individual members of a ward team will never be fully competent. This is where the three levels of competence suggested by the RCN ('competent', 'experienced' and 'senior practitioner') become relevant. Furthermore, the concept of 'team competence' (previously probably best known as 'skill mix') protects individual practitioners as they advance, adjust or expand their practice through the skills/career trajectory. In this sense, the team members have a responsibility to support each other to develop practice. The team structure also prevents nurse-facilitated discharge from remaining the domain of a select few.

Implementing a competency framework for discharge

Competency framework

A competency framework for discharge practice should be implemented through a systematic replicable process (Lees & Emmerson 2006). This implementation process involves four key elements:

1. Plan the education required

2. Develop discharge skills in practice (applied behaviour)

3. Develop nurse-facilitated discharge (use skills and knowledge actively)

4. Audit and research developments (engaging staff for future)

The majority of competencies already established are specific in terms of 'what' has to be achieved. Yet they are relatively high-level, and generally lacking in detailed guidance on 'how' they are to be achieved and over what timescale. The successful implementation of competencies requires a wide range of flexible learning opportunities and techniques to suit individual learning styles (Williams 2003). For instance, busy practitioners need support in practice from expert facilitation to develop knowledge, skills and competencies in order to perform new multi-professional roles (Bharr 1998, Jones 1999). The box below offers an overview of how competency in blood result interpretation might be achieved. This is cited as one of the six competencies needed for nurse-facilitated discharge (see Chapter 3).

Background and theory

Achieving competency

Achieving competency in blood results interpretation

Stages involved (6)

1. Attendance at one lead lecture set at post-registration level for 'experienced nurses' (see RCN reference). Read and understand underpinning information sources related to blood results.

(Learning objective: to gain prerequisite baseline knowledge regarding commonly requested blood investigations)

2. Participation in the process of reporting blood results received in your practice area by separating blood results into:
    A. Results within universally accepted normal ranges
    B. Results outside universally accepted normal ranges

(Learning objective: to participate in the process and familiarise yourself with results received, which may be outside normal range)

3. Participate in a ward round where the patient's results are discussed in the context of the overall patient condition/diagnosis/working diagnosis. Alternatively, if a ward round is not taking place, conduct a discussion with a member of the consultant's medical team.

(Learning objective: to begin to apply knowledge and results together; to further personal understanding of appropriate connections between diagnosis, treatment and nursing care required)

4. Complete continual professional development document (CPD) with case studies, participating in reflective practice.

(Learning objective: to document evidence of 'on the job learning' that has taken place and identify areas for further development required)

5. Proactively network with other colleagues also undertaking this programme of learning related to blood results reporting, by feeding back learning at a ward teaching session with peers.

(Learning objective: to build confidence in your own decision-making and reporting skills and provide a feedback loop for discussion of pertinent issues arising)

6. Participation in oral discussion with senior level doctor in area of blood results, reporting pertinent to role and subsequent declaration of competence through completed competency document.

(Learning objective: to accept responsibility for level of competency achieved and acknowledge 'lifelong learning for other areas of practice')

Assessing and maintaining competency

When the experiential learning is completed, competencies need to be assessed. This should not be approached as a subjective self-assessment or 'tick box' exercise, adding to the pile of meaningless paper in a dusty portfolio. On the contrary, competencies should be transparent, interactive, live and constantly evolving.

Implementation of competencies can potentially open up a can of worms, highlighting the huge responsibility that needs to be embraced, shared and sustained by employees/employers alike. For example, following the development of competence, staff will still need support (time out) for the updating/maintenance and adjustment of competence, bearing in mind that practice does not remain static.

Moreover, foundation work, such as undertaking a training needs analysis, which supports competence, may not have been systematically developed in the first place. In this case, remedial action would be required before competency development can be fully undertaken. It should also be remembered that education and subsequent competencies are only part of the story. Training also needs to interface with clinical supervision and governance plans in order to reduce clinical risks and improve the quality of patient care. Competencies are a vehicle to support and protect practitioners as they gain confidence in developing holistic new areas of practice.

Other approaches to discharge training

The greater the range of skills development approaches employed, the more likely any programme is to be sustainable in the longer term. For example, traditional didactic learning approaches have become rather outmoded, with today's sharp focus on delivering results in the workplace. Staff members from different professional backgrounds are now being encouraged to acquire skills and competencies in a flexible manner.

Five approaches are suggested:
1. Staff rotations (experiential learning)
2. Undertaking non-clinical existing learning opportunities (agreed as part of the Knowledge and Skills Framework)

3. Undertaking formal education at universities
   (Didactic/academic)
4. Secondments to gain specific skills or experience as a stepping stone into new roles
5. Completion of new clinical skills as part of sets (to be accredited as Credit Accumulated Transfer Schemes in the future)

Skill sets

Skill sets

To aid cohesive nurse facilitation of the plethora of services that exist to support discharging patients from hospital, 'skill sets' could be established. These would group together the particular competencies, skills required (if competencies are not yet developed) and training opportunities into a set, which addresses all the patient's needs. While individual skills can be learned through supplementary approaches, these are best applied holistically to patient care. Otherwise, there is a danger of creating a task-orientated approach where skills do not join up to benefit the patient, especially those related to specialist areas of practice.

A discharge planning skill set may therefore require the inclusion of supplementary competencies that are not traditionally associated with discharge planning. For example, as services become more cosmopolitan, spanning boundaries, discharge may equate to 'transfer of care' (where patients are transferred into other services). In such cases, knowledge of other interfacing services will be vital.

A skill set needed for nurse-facilitated discharge of an older person is shown as an example in the box below. This skill set may typically comprise: knowledge, comprehension, application and evaluation throughout services, and pertinent assessments leading to referrals/good liaison abilities (which should not be taken for granted).

Although there are many good ideas on how to impart new skills, successful implementation is often constrained because there is no consistent approach to skills development throughout the organisation. It would therefore be helpful if access points into skill sets could be introduced at the point of recruitment. This would replace the present ad hoc approach with a more gradual progression, in which the study time required for each person would be fairly apportioned as necessary. To promote professional growth of individual staff members, it is also essential to determine what knowledge, skills and experience in discharge planning they possess on arrival. If this initial assessment does not take place, their skills and abilities may not be effectively utilised from the outset of employment, and stagnation or regression may occur.

Required skill set

Skill set needed for nurse-facilitated discharge of an older person

(This skill set would be needed in addition to the six core competencies described in Chapter 3.)

- Knowledge of mechanisms that explain the process to patients and their carers
- Understanding of services available for older people
- Demonstrable knowledge of intermediate care and social care services
- Understanding of chronic disease management
- Understanding of the tools available to assist discharge planning
- Good communication, liaison and documentation skills
- Completing the Single Assessment Process
- Conducting a range of relevant assessments: social, falls, frailty, abbreviated mental test scoring
- Making simple referrals (e.g. to district nursing, transport requests, etc.)
- Engaging voluntary services and patient representatives
- Making appropriate referrals to intermediate care services
- Making referral to social care services for instigation or restarting of services
- Making referral to Elderly Care Assessment Unit
- Submitting a Section (2) and (5) form
- Following up of patients

Background and theory

Implementing nurse-facilitated discharge

The specific processes and tools for implementing nurse-facilitated discharge are discussed in Chapter 5 ('Instigating and maintaining the strategic momentum'). The case studies in Section 3 provide further reinforcement of the overall concept, particularly the leading case study 'protocol or bespoke'. In summary, any of the methods outlined below can be utilised to drive nurse-facilitated discharge practice forward, as long as there is clarity about the method being used.

These methods are:

- Using bespoke discharge management plans (useful in emergency admissions)
- Writing discharge checklists with variance measured against the norm (day surgery)
- Protocol or criteria-driven discharges (useful for specific condition groups)
- Care pathways with integrated discharge points (for specific operations of procedures spanning different organisations delivering care)

No single approach to implementing nurse-facilitated discharges will be appropriate across a whole organisation. To some extent, the approach selected will depend upon organisational readiness and the particular area of practice. For example, Trauma and Orthopaedics, General Surgery and Gynaecology were the first areas to express an interest in developing systems to support nurses in facilitating discharge. In each case, while the discharge process was clearly stated as part of a care pathway, detailed work was still required to specify 'how' it should be carried out. In some instances, this required the drawing up of a protocol, with discharge parameters aligned to the greater majority of patients with a particular condition or following a particular procedure/operation.

In contrast, acute medical patients may be affected by many variables, which make it difficult to use a protocol-managed approach to their discharge. In this case, a criteria-led approach, with the post-take ward round providing a management plan and estimated date of discharge, may be far more appropriate. Furthermore, the management plan in itself may encourage a reductionist approach, whereby the nurse may be tempted to rely on the plan alone (in a rapidly changing acute environment). The nurse may not then use other tools that are available, such as the Single Assessment Process or other assessments that have been carried out since admission.

Regardless of the approach used, it is worth remembering that patients enter into a process once they are admitted to hospital. The discharge should always be viewed as part of this process, rather than a single unconnected task or checklist.

Patient involvement in discharge

Patient involvement

Without doubt, the relationship between the nurse and the patients they care for is central to the success of nurse-facilitated discharge. Increasingly, nurses are being asked to adopt practices that provide evidence of patients' involvement in their own care. Many supporting systems are evolving, and some have always been better than others. Patient notice boards (by the bed), patient information leaflets, patient focus groups and satisfaction surveys have become commonplace.

In complex discharges, the patient's involvement has always been a pivotal part of the discharge liaison nurse's role. Even in simple discharges there should be varying degrees of patient involvement. However, these are often cursory or superficial, and there is a long way to go in order to develop relationships that truly achieve patient empowerment (Brown *et al.* 2006).

Evidence of patient involvement in the discharge plan is required (DoH 2005c, CNST: DoH 2003a) and this can be achieved in its simplest form through meaningful conversations that are documented in the patient's records. Chronic disease management and admission prevention through case management and new roles in the community also play an important part in discharge planning. The promotion of self-care strategies is a distinct and evolving part of the nurse's role (DoH 2005c).

None of these are new concepts, but they may need to be given a higher profile in discharge planning. If all these aspects are effectively brought together they will certainly help to give patient involvement a more central position in discharge planning. Some further practical tips for nurses on increasing patient involvement in discharge are offered below as examples:

- Identify how you can help your patients learn from each other.
- Involve patients in their discharge plans.
- Provide patients with regular information.
- A nursing presence on the ward round reinforces good communication with the patient.
- Arrange meetings with the family and carers, taking time to meet during visiting periods.
- Involve patients when completing their discharge checklist.
- Give a clear estimate of date of discharge as soon after admission as is practical.
- Guide doctors and other professionals on ways of increasing patient involvement.

All sorts of impressive plans can be made by professionals but if they have not been discussed or shared with the patient they are not likely to be executed with any success.

Conclusion

At present, discharge planning has a very high profile across the NHS, with systems and practices constantly playing catch-up in their attempts to integrate policy into practice settings. Nurse-facilitated discharge from hospital is multifaceted. I feel we are at the beginning of something very great in the history of nursing. The time is right to bring about these changes, along with many other new ways of working, to support far-reaching developments in the NHS.

At the very least, we should be able to look back in future years and see, irrespective of the exact terminology used to frame the policy, that nurse-facilitated discharge has improved care for our patients. To succeed, it requires many different healthcare professionals to draw on their own experience and share it with each other, creating a truly integrated approach, both professionally and organisationally, in the best interests of the patient.

This book offers three perspectives to illuminate this vast subject. Section 1 discusses the theoretical aspects, Section 2 covers clinical practice considerations, and Section 3 offers case examples from practitioners, to whom all the credit in interpreting the changes, and facing the challenges, should rightly be given.

References

Atwal, A. (2002). 'Nurses' perceptions of discharge planning in acute health care: a case study in one British teaching hospital'. *Journal of Advanced Nursing,* 39 (5), 450–458.

Bargargliotti, T., Luttrell, M. & Lenburg, C. (1999). 'Reducing threats to the implementation of a competency-based performance assessment system'. *Journal of Issues in Nursing.* (www.nursingworld.org)

Barr, H. (1998). 'Competent to collaborate: towards a competency-based model for inter-professional education'. *Journal of Interprofessional Care,* 12 (2), 181.

Brown, D., McWilliam, C. & Ward-Griffin, C. (2006). 'Client-centred empowering partnership in nursing'. *Journal of Advanced Nursing,* 53 (2), 160–168.

Department of Health (2000). 'The NHS Plan: a plan for improvement, a plan for reform'. London: The Stationery Office.

Department of Health (2001a). 'The National Service Framework for Older People'. London: The Stationery Office.

Department of Health (2001b). 'The single assessment process consultation papers and process: an introduction to single assessment'. London: The Stationery Office.

Department of Health (2002a). 'Discharge planning: model discharge documentation'. London: The Stationery Office.

Department of Health (2002b). Health and Social Care Joint Unit and Change Agent Team, 'Discharge from Hospital: a good practice checklist'. London: The Stationery Office. (www.dh.gov.uk/assetRoot/04/12/62/50/04126250.pdf)

Department of Health & Royal College of Nursing (2003). 'The Freedom to Practise: dispelling the myths'. London: The Stationery Office.

Department of Health (2003a). 'Effectiveness of inpatient discharge procedure'. London: The Stationery Office.

Department of Health (2003b). 'Discharge from Hospital: pathway, process and practice'. London: The Stationery Office.

Department of Health (2003c). 'Making amends: proposals for clinical negligence reforms'. London: The Stationery Office.

Department of Health (2003d). 'The community care (delayed discharges) act LAC/2003 guidance for implementation'. London: The Stationery Office.

Department of Health (2004a). 'Achieving timely "simple" discharge from hospital: A toolkit for the multidisciplinary team'. London: The Stationery Office.

Background and theory

Department of Health (2004b). 'The NHS Knowledge and Skills Framework (NHS KSF) and the Development Review process'. London: The Stationery Office.

Department of Health (2005a). 'Creating a patient-led NHS: delivering the improvement plan'. London: The Stationery Office.

Department of Health (2005b). 'Commissioning a patient-led NHS'. London: The Stationery Office.

Department of Health (2005c). 'Supporting people with long-term conditions: liberating the talents of nursing, caring for people with long-term conditions'. London: The Stationery Office.

Efraimsson, E., Rasmussen, B., Gilje, F. & Sandman, P. (2003). 'Expressions of power and powerlessness in discharge planning: a case study of an older woman on her way home'. *Journal of Clinical Nursing*, 12 (5), 707–716.

Jones, A. (1999). 'The place of judgement in competency-based assessment'. *Journal of Vocational Education and Training*. 51 (1), 145–160.

Kuockkanen, L. & Leino-Kilpi (2000). 'Power and empowerment in nursing: three theoretical approaches'. *Journal of Advanced Nursing*, 31 (1), 235–241.

Leason, K. (2003). 'Delay tactics'. *Nursing Standard*, 17 (24), 16–17.

Lees, L. (2004). 'Making nurse-led discharge work to improve patient care'. *Nursing Times*, 100 (37), 30–32. (www.nursingtimes.net)

Lees, L. (2006a). 'Not Just another sheet of paper: discharge checklists'. *The Communicator*, RCN discharge planning and continuing care forum, Summer 2006, 4–5. www.rcn.org.uk/liaisondischarge

Lees, L. (2006b). 'Emergency Care Briefing Paper: Modernising discharge from hospital', updated version, January 2006. National Electronic Library for Health, 3,100 words and 62 references. (http://libraries.nelh.nhs.uk/emergency/viewResource.asp?uri = http%3A//libraries.nelh.nhs.uk/common/resources/%3Fid%3D63696&categoryID = 1414)

Lees, L. & Holmes, C. (2005). 'Estimating date of discharge at ward level: a pilot study'. *Nursing Standard*, 19 (17), 40–43.

Lees, L., Allen, G. & O'Brien, D. (2006). 'Using post-take ward rounds to facilitate simple discharge'. *Nursing Times*, 102 (18), 28–30. (www.nursingtimes.net)

Lees, L. & Emmerson, K. (2006). 'Identifying discharge practice training needs'. *Nursing Standard*, 20 (29), 47–51. (www.nursing-standard.co.uk)

National Audit Office (2003). 'Ensuring the effective discharge of older patients from NHS acute hospitals'. London: The Stationery Office.

Nursing and Midwifery Council (2004). 'The NMC Code of Professional Conduct: standards for conduct, performance and ethics'. London: Nursing and Midwifery Council.

Pethybridge, J. (2004). 'How team working influences discharge planning from hospital: a study of four multidisciplinary teams in an acute hospital in England'. *Journal of Interprofessional Care*, **18** (1), 29–41.

Royal College of Nursing (2006). 'Core Career and Competency Framework'. (www.rcn.org.uk/resources/corecompetences)

Rudd, C. & Smith, J. (2002). 'Discharge planning'. *Nursing Standard*, **17** (5), 33–37.

Rushforth, H. & Glasper, E.A. (1999). 'Implications of nursing role expansion for professional practice'. *British Journal of Nursing*, **8** (22).

Williams, M. (2003). 'Assessment of portfolios in professional education'. *Nursing Standard*, **18** (8), 33–37.

Chapter 2

Developing nurse-facilitated discharge policy and its interface with healthcare practice

Tracey Riley

This chapter will discuss some of the issues that frequently arise within NHS organisations, as national policy on discharge planning is interpreted and implemented in practice settings.

Establishing the nurse's role in facilitating discharge presents many challenges for individual practitioners providing care. First, the practitioners themselves are at the sharp edge of any new ways of working, and they may often be unprepared for, and unconvinced by, the need for change. Frequently asked questions need to be addressed and resolved before successful change can take place. These questions may include:

- Is this change for change's sake?
- How will these changes impact on my workload, which is already heavy?
- What support will I receive?
- Will this extension of my role be rewarded by professional recognition or be reflected in my salary?

Change must be managed effectively, and preparation, planning and discussion are crucial to ensure success. This is particularly important at a time when change is occurring across the whole of the NHS, with differing priorities and agendas causing tensions at practice level and beyond.

Admission and discharge

Admission is described as inappropriate when there are suitable alternatives available (DoH 2004a). These alternatives may involve accessing the relevant care or ensuring that the patient's needs are met at home. In 2004, the Department of Health issued a good practice guide (DoH 2004b) to prevent admission or reduce the length of stay in hospital. This guide included examples of techniques such as pre-screening, assessment and establishing a framework of support.

Bed days in hospital are expensive and the measures outlined in the above document are partly a response to work done by the Audit Commission (2002). The Audit Commission suggests that the 'vicious cycle' of readmission for chronic and long-term conditions can be replaced by a 'virtuous cycle' that prevents early discharge because of pressure on beds. Vetter (2003) suggests that a lack of definition of the discharge planning concept and poor measurement tools add to the problem of patients being discharged and promptly readmitted, particularly in view of the rapidly increasing demand from patients and the diminishing supply of beds.

Instead, Rudd (2002) states that the focus should be on careful assessment and screening, and that discharge planning should begin as soon as the decision to admit a patient has been made. The complex nature of the many interlinking policies concerned, makes effective nurse-facilitated discharge even more important in the wider NHS context.

Why should nurses facilitate appropriate discharge?

Why nurses?

Nurses are ideally placed to facilitate appropriate discharge of patients for several reasons (DoH 2000). First, nurses quickly develop relationships with their patients, both therapeutically and personally, because they spend more time with patients than any other professional group. Secondly, nurses are increasingly advancing their role and status within the multidisciplinary team. It therefore makes sense for them to use their extended skills and knowledge base to develop a personalised discharge package, after consultation with the patient and other professionals.

The NHS Plan and 'Ten key roles for nurses' (DoH 2000) gave nurses particular responsibility for the admission and discharge of patients living with specific conditions and whose circumstances could be managed within the agreed protocols.

Brown *et al.* (2006) report on a study that looked at nurses' attitudes to client empowerment one year after implementing client-centred care in a practice setting. The metaphor used to describe the nurses' changing attitudes was that of Dorothy's journey in *The Wizard of Oz* (Baum 1963). The nurses' experience began with them becoming aware of profound change. They then encountered disempowering barriers, and finally learnt from the experience to complete their journey towards client-centred empowerment.

Specific training challenges

Training challenges

Policy challenges present themselves as practitioners encounter a change in working practice that requires a revision of their skills and knowledge base. Active management of discharge planning requires nurses to juggle competing priorities and patient needs, and a toolkit exists to help them make these decisions (DoH 2004c).

'The NHS Knowledge and Skills Framework' (DoH 2004b) outlines the knowledge and skills required for a range of expanded roles and nurse-led practices. Self-assessment of training needs can sometimes be an uncomfortable process, especially if there is limited self-awareness and the picture that emerges is different from the one the practitioner expected (Lees & Emmerson 2006).

In addition, the learning curve for practitioners may be very steep at first. The resources needed to carry out such extensive training can place a burden on budgets and staffing levels. This obvious cause of strain at practice level should be acknowledged and addressed. Nurses need to meet the challenge of developing their range of skills and extending their practice beyond previously acknowledged boundaries. Likewise, those responsible for policing the standards of advanced nursing roles have to rise to the challenge of ensuring that appropriate training is provided.

Lees and Emmerson (2006) say that specific training should take place so that nurses are prepared for any extension of their existing role. They add that nurses need to have some formalisation of 'on the job' learning, and this depends on them having an effective learning environment. However, an overly formal learning process can make the experience stressful and this may detract from its value. Another approach may be to encourage reflection within a clinical supervision context so that practitioners can explore their own progress with honesty. A reflective diary will help track progress made and identify any issues that arise. This will enable nurses to map their own journey towards enhanced practice.

Yet how do we promote new practice when staff members are often under so much pressure to meet basic care demands? And does the success of this process influence the formation of policy at a higher level? Davies (2004) argues that nursing voices are afforded little respect in political debate, and suggests that nursing leaders should acknowledge the complex position that nurses occupy in healthcare. Nurses have traditionally presented themselves as the champions of the patient. In view of this, perhaps the increasing profile of patient groups will provide nurses with more of a platform on the political stage.

Understanding policy at practice level

Policy at practice level

Nurses working at an operational, practice level need to understand both the vertical dimension of policy formation and the horizontal dimension of policy implementation in order to appreciate the complexity of the change needed. This understanding elevates the new policy's relevance, and gives it worth and sustainability (Colebatch 2002). According to Colebatch, the horizontal dimensions concern relationships between policy participants in different hospital departments. It is also essential to consider existing national policies, and the different agendas and priorities being presented at local level.

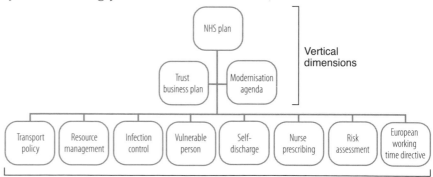

Vertical and horizontal dimensions of policy

The above diagram illustrates some of the vertical and horizontal dimensions of policy. It demonstrates how the vertical (strategic) dimensions influence and impact upon the horizontal dimensions, which are more readily considered by practitioners at an operational level.

Problems to solve, or dilemmas to manage?

Problem or dilemma?

It is necessary to look at the difference between problems to solve and dilemmas to manage, as illustrated in Johnson's (1996) description of polarity management. When a dilemma has been identified, the two opposing potential solutions need to be explored. By addressing the positive and negative aspects of these two solutions, each quadrant can be explored in depth, giving a fuller picture of the situation. Johnson (1996) advises that when investigating each quadrant it is helpful to use a structure to 'frame' the quadrants. The table below shows, as an example, the opposing arguments on the subject of nurses extending roles and expanding skills. Here, the positive and negative aspects of both poles are considered. Those involved are invited to contribute to whichever viewpoint they currently hold, on the understanding that they will hear and consider the other standpoints and argument

L+	R+
● More responsive to patient needs ● Care is seamless and timely ● Nurses experience empowerment ● Job satisfaction and sense of value increase as role grows ● Wider role and responsibility enables more holistic approach ● Encourages innovation and improvement	● Nurses stay within their comfort zone ● Workload is predictable and routine ● Practice safe in the knowledge that others are of similar standard and ability ● Belief that there is more 'bedside' time ● Non-threatening environment
Extended/Expanded role and skills	Traditional role and skills
L−	R−
● Having enough to do already ● What if something goes wrong? ● Achieving/proving competence ● Nursing should stay at the 'bedside' ● Nurses not deemed competent may believe themselves fit for purpose and pose a danger	● Practice becomes stagnant and automatic ● Patient may experience delays in treatment by appropriate professional ● Less professional opportunity ● Nurses at times rendered 'powerless' until appropriate professional intervenes

Background and theory

Encouraging stakeholders to examine other standpoints will provide them with a valuable insight into the multi-dimensional process of formulating agendas and priorities. This culture of openness should make the change easier to cope with, and gaining an appreciation of the wider picture will help relieve some of the worry that practitioners feel when faced with change.

Bacchi (1991) advocates a 'What's the problem?' question approach when considering policy formation. Here we can consider, for instance, whether the introduction of a nurse-led care policy is in response to the question: 'What can we do to improve patients' experience of ill-health, in terms of providing access to help in crisis situations?' Alternatively, a nurse-led care policy could be a response to the question: 'What can we do to save money and reduce the impact of impending financial crisis?'

This example illustrates the multi-faceted nature of policy, not just at its inception but throughout the process of implementation and beyond. Taking a 'What's the problem?' approach helps us to understand the complex relationships and conflicts between established policies and priorities. Stone (2002, p. 156) says that, because of these complexities, it may not be possible to examine policy formation using standard logical analysis. It is difficult to take an objective approach to what is effectively a collection of subjective opinions, beliefs and agendas. For example, broad national agendas must co-exist with the narrower, interlinking policies and protocols that are already in place at local level.

Overcoming barriers to change

Barriers to change

Other professionals from the multidisciplinary team need to be included in the creation of new policy, as nurses cannot implement and manage all the change required on their own (Hancock & Campbell 2006). It is essential to develop an appreciation of all the dimensions involved. However, even if professional boundaries and responsibilities merge and blur, the patient must always remain the central focus of the policy.

Patients rarely see only one professional group. They are often referred for expert opinion or treatment to several groups. Clear channels of communication are therefore needed to avoid repetition, oversight and professional rivalry. At practice level, it is necessary to reconcile the differences that stand as potential barriers to success at the interface between policy and practice and this is more readily achieved with an open mind and a willingness to hear the other side of the argument and explore the subject with a spirit of open-ended enquiry. The common value must be the best interests of the patient/client.

There are also issues of accountability and competence. Ensuring that practitioners are fit for purpose is a challenge, which requires strong leadership and effective monitoring of practice standards. Again, polarity management is a useful tool to manage these tensions, as it encourages practitioners to look at the wider picture. Stone (2002) suggests that conflict over minor details is a sign that the fundamental story needs clarifying.

Asking the big questions will prevent the automatic response of papering over the cracks while ignoring major issues. In any case, until the larger problems are dealt with, the minor problems will keep resurfacing elsewhere.

Change is a complex process and Nemeth (2003) advises that communication, leadership, coordination of activities and integration of the changes into practice patterns are essential to achieve positive outcomes. Deegan (2005) suggests that an individual should be identified as the agent of change. This person then needs to choose, develop and order the activities needed to bring about change. However, it could be argued that formalising the change process in this way could make practitioners wary and sceptical. Gradual, evolutionary change may be more acceptable in some areas. Whichever approach is taken, effective change management is essential so that practitioners can ask questions, and feel they are being heard and valued.

Conclusion

The vast majority of nurses find themselves at the policy–practice interface, implementing rather than influencing policy. The need to develop a comprehensive policy stream for multiple users within the multidisciplinary team is an important aspect of planning, implementation and working within the policy as a process. Practitioners involved in the patient's care journey should be able to access a comprehensive patient history or record to facilitate seamless care.

Background and theory

While policy forms a central part of the national modernisation agenda, it is vital to maintain a focus on the contextual factors and recognise their importance. Ultimately, policy is a process and is not fixed or rigid. Policy responds to change as much as change is affected by policy. Like practice itself, policy should remain fluid, responsive and patient-centred.

References

Audit Commission (2002). 'Integrated services for older people'.
London: The Stationery Office.

Bacchi, C.L. (1999). *Women, policy and politics: the construction of policy problems.* London: Sage.

Baum, L.F. (1963). *The Wizard of Oz.* New York: Grosset and Dunlap.

Brown, D., McWilliam, C. & Ward-Griffin, C. (2006). 'Client-centred empowering partnership in nursing'. *Journal of Advanced Nursing,* 53 (2), 160–168.

Colebatch, H.K. (2002). 'Who makes policy', in *Policy* (2nd edn). Buckingham: Open University Press, 22–37.

Davies, C. (2004). 'Political leadership and the politics of nursing'. *Journal of Nursing Management,* 12, 235–241.

Deegan, C., Watson, A., Nestor, G., Conlon, C., & Connaughton, F. (2005). 'Managing change initiatives in clinical areas'. *Nursing Management,* 12 (4), July, 24–29.

Department of Health (2000). 'Developing key roles for nurses and midwives: A guide for managers'. London: The Stationery Office.

Department of Health (2004a). 'Avoiding and diverting admissions to hospital – a good practice guide'. London: The Stationery Office.

Department of Health (2004b). 'The NHS Knowledge and Skills Framework (NHS KSF) and the Development Review Process'.
London: The Stationery Office.

Department of Health (2004c). 'Achieving timely "simple" discharge from hospital: A toolkit for the multidisciplinary team'. London: The Stationery Office.

Hancock, H. & Campbell, S. (2006). 'Impact of leading an empowered organisation programme'. *Nursing Standard,* 20 (19), 41–48.

Johnson, B. (1996). 'Teamwork is not a solution' in *Polarity Management: Identifying and managing unsolvable problems.* Mass: HRD Press, 3–17.

Lees, L. & Emmerson, K. (2006). 'Identifying discharge practice training needs'. *Nursing Standard,* 20 (29), 47–51.

Nemeth, L. (2003). 'Implementing change for effective outcomes'. *Outcomes Management,* 7 (3), July/Sep, 134–139.

Rudd, C. (2002). 'Discharge planning'. *Nursing Standard,* 17 (5), 33–37.

Background and theory

Stone, D. (2002). 'Symbols' in *Policy paradox: the art of political decision making* (2nd edn). New York: W.W. Norton and Company.

Vetter, N. (2003). 'Inappropriately delayed discharge from hospital: What do we know?' *British Medical Journal*, 326, 927–928.

Chapter 3

Educational support for discharge planning

Ann Saxon

This chapter will explore creative and innovative ways of delivering education and training in discharge planning. Learning involves embracing the process of change (Reece & Walker 2003, p. 59), both by gaining a better understanding of our own experiences and by moving through spectrums of personal growth. Learning about discharge planning through innovative education gives practitioners an opportunity to engage in a collaborative approach to learning, and also enables them to apply their newly acquired skills in practice.

Teaching is not only about designing educational packages. The teacher should not merely be seen as a purveyor of knowledge (Reece & Walker 2004, p. 3) but also as a facilitator: someone who helps students to learn for themselves. Designing innovative educational materials for effective discharge planning should create an opportunity for enhanced inter-professional collaboration. This should increase learning by allowing practitioners to share their experiences. It should also enable them to become more self-directed as learners.

In the current political climate, discharge planning is high on the agenda for all healthcare organisations. The creation of any educational materials for healthcare practitioners should be informed by current sociological, political, professional and personal knowledge of the factors influencing discharge planning. The effects on patients and their carers (whether simple or complex care packages are required) must also be taken into account.

The main considerations in developing educational materials for discharge planning are therefore:

Background and theory

- Current policy: national service frameworks, legislation, patient service agreements
- Epidemiology: chronic disease
- Sociological perspective: demographics, ageing population, disability, long-term conditions
- Professional knowledge: key skills, competency, role development, inter-professional working, leadership

The National Health Service (NHS) is ever changing. Education must keep pace so that it can be proactive instead of simply reacting to change. It is therefore essential in designing any educational materials for healthcare practitioners that all of the above factors are considered and implemented throughout.

The educational arena

Educational arena

Training for professional practice usually requires the learner to follow a particular syllabus laid down by a governing body such as the Nursing and Midwifery Council (NMC) or the Health Professions Council (HPC). These awarding bodies for professional practice set minimum standards, which have to be explicitly set out in any curriculum. When developing new course materials and educational packages it is advisable to check the most up-to-date published standards. These can usually be found on the professional bodies' websites (for example www.nmc.org.uk and www.qaa.ac.uk).

The Quality Assurance Agency for Higher Education (QAA) is the governing body that oversees the development of professional courses in higher education institutions (HEI). The QAA was established in 1997 to monitor the quality of standards for professional practice, and to provide an integrated quality assurance service for higher education in the UK. In reviewing academic standards, they can describe the level of achievement a student has reached to gain an academic award such as a degree. To demonstrate the required standards, the QAA have developed subject benchmark statements that identify the expected outcomes of a particular degree in a particular subject. When designing any new courses, it is advisable to match course content to the subject specialist benchmark statement. The QAA has also set up a code of practice.(www.qaa.ac.uk/aboutus/qaaIntro/intro.asp).

The use of e-learning

e-learning

E-learning has been around in some form since the development of the computer (Shank & Sitze 2004). It can be in the form of interactive material via a CD-Rom or other medium. This also includes online learning, which is the use of network technologies such as the internet for delivering and assessing a range of materials. Online learning will be discussed later in this chapter (see p. 43).

E-learning materials should follow guidelines to ensure that they have been designed in the most effective way for students to use, following recommendations from the Higher Education Funding Council Executive (HEFCE). It is also important to consider the special educational needs of students and the policy in place to support and protect learners with disabilities (SENDA 2001). In the Government's white paper 'The Future of Higher Education' (DfES 2004), the Higher Education Funding Council is charged with ensuring that e-learning is embedded in training/educational programmes in a full and sustainable way. They suggest that an e-learning strategy should embrace:

1. The internet and use of new technologies
2. New approaches to learning and teaching (including work-placed learning and blended learning) that are emerging in response to diverse student and employer demand
3. The opportunities offered by wholly internet-based learning to explore exciting technological approaches and to provide global delivery (HEFC 2004, www.hefc.ac.uk)

Designing new training courses

Designing training

There are many aspects of policy and practice that should be taken into account when designing training courses for discharge planning practice. Although nurses in a ward environment may have the most day-to-day contact with patients, many other professionals will also be involved. It is therefore important to adopt an inter-professional approach to planning a new curriculum or course. This will encourage the development of a range of skills in order to complement the roles of different professional groups. It will also ultimately benefit patients and carers by giving them access to a range of health professionals who should be able to ensure more efficient and effective hospital discharge (DoH 2004).

New methods of delivering training need to be developed in order to ensure that courses meet the needs of twenty-first century practitioners. The next part of this chapter will explore the methods being used to modernise education.

Modernising education

Modernising education

Modernising education has been on the agenda in recent years for many professional groups – not only healthcare practitioners. Patients and carers can access information more easily nowadays, and their expectations of care are far higher than in the past. Developing a wide repertoire of new skills in discharge planning could be a way of meeting the expectations and needs expressed by patients.

Bradshaw (1972), cited in Harris,A. (1997), put forward the following taxonomy of need:

- Felt need: gap between knowledge and practice
- Expressed need: new programme needs development
- Unmet need: no new programmes exist

This taxonomy can be applied to learners and teachers in relation to modernising education. It could also be used in marketing new courses, to show how they have been developed to meet particular needs.

Previous educational programmes relied heavily on the learner being a passive recipient of knowledge and the teacher being considered the expert (Reece & Walker 2004). Nursing education programmes used to focus mainly on the input of knowledge without considering the changes that take place in the individual who has undergone new learning. Sometimes it is only long after the learner has completed a course that the real benefits of that learning can be measured.

Students often recall what they have learnt when they can apply it to an actual situation that they find themselves in. For example, it is hard to appreciate the importance of developing discharge planning skills when learning them in a classroom. It is only when the practitioner is called upon to use the new skills in practice that their importance is truly understood.

Educational support for discharge planning

Most healthcare undergraduate programmes now deliver innovative, dynamic courses in many areas ranging from change management to leadership development. Examples of the diverse training approaches used include:

- Problem-based learning
- Reflective practice
- Virtual learning communities
- Online learning
- Clinical practice assimilation

Some of these will now be explored in more detail.

Problem-based learning

Problem-based learning

Problem-based learning has its origins in several schools of philosophical thought, mainly those of naturalism, metaphysics, phenomenology and rationalism (Howell Major & Savin-Baden 2004). This approach encourages learners to make sense of situations, such as planning a patient's discharge from hospital in a reasoned, logical way. In simple terms, problem-based learning encourages students to break down an apparently complex situation, and then analyse the causes that led to the situation, and the factors influencing people's thoughts, feelings and behaviours in the situation.

Problem-based learning is a complex approach and should include all the learning that is required as well as the assessment of that learning in a supported and facilitated way. Some of the advantages offered by problem-based learning have been described by Weller (2002, p. 71). These include:

- Increased student motivation
- Development of problem-solving skills
- Increased student responsibility
- Flexibility
- Exposure to different ideas and solutions
- Contextualisation of information
- Interactive and engaging
- Deepening of the skills of reflection and analysis

Online learning

Online learning

Online learning has become very popular because it allows learners to access information and courses wherever and whenever they can. Staff working in any healthcare context need education to be as accessible as possible. Although time is set aside to attend mandatory courses, non-mandatory courses are usually less well attended, unless they form part of a more formal award such as a first degree or master's degree. Online facilities open up a wealth of opportunities for all types of students including those working part-time or during the early evening or at night. According to Shank and Sitze (2004, p. 2), 'Online learning involves the use of network technologies (such as the internet and business networks) for delivering, supporting and assessing formal and informal instruction.'

They go on to say that this type of learning may utilise many online resources and materials, including electronic libraries, learning materials and courses, real-time and non-real-time discussion forums and conferencing, and knowledge-sharing forums.

Despite the many positive aspects of online learning, a note of warning should be sounded that some online materials may not be of sufficiently high quality. In addition, some online courses may not be recognised by professional accreditation bodies. Nevertheless, for employers who are finding it difficult to release staff for training away from the workplace, online learning may offer a useful form of training within the working environment. Finally, employers increasingly require proof that learning is making a difference in practice. It is often time-consuming and not cost-effective to release staff for traditional courses. Online learning, in contrast, can be scheduled into the working day, making it more accessible and cost-effective. Staff could work towards projects and plans required for the development of the organisation.

Other factors to consider when using online materials are:

- Accessibility of computer equipment
- Accessibility of network
- Confidence of learner in using computers
- Copyright material (owners of the online material own the copyright so it would be important to check ownership of material before use)
- Reviewed material (information available online may not always have been reviewed and this needs to be taken into consideration when using such sources)
- Accreditation of course/academic currency
- Cost

Developing effective training partnerships

It is essential to have effective partnerships between educational establishments and practice areas when developing new training courses. These partnerships can be formed in different ways. One approach is through the validation and accreditation of formal programmes such as initial entry nursing programmes, which require 50 per cent of the course to be supported in practice settings.

Less formally, a partnership can be created by means of clinical practitioners working alongside educationalists in research or development. For example, the university lecturer may be very important in interpreting a practitioner's view, from the pragmatic aspects to achieving theoretical outcomes of a programme or course. If there is a sound relationship, university staff can play a valuable role in guiding practitioners through the sometimes difficult process of getting courses validated and accredited.

The development of a specific discharge training module

The next part of this chapter will discuss how such a partnership can be helpful in designing new materials in an innovative and creative way. It will outline how a local university worked collaboratively with a Foundation Trust Hospital to develop a course for health professionals in effective discharge planning.

The impetus to develop the course came from a senior lecturer working in the School of Primary Health Care, Faculty of Health, at the University of Central England (UCE) in Birmingham, and a consultant nurse working in acute medicine at a local Foundation Hospital Trust. In working together, the need for a particular course related to discharge planning became evident.

Identifying the need for training and assessing the cost

One of the aspects noted was that student nurses appeared to have very little knowledge of the discharge process. On taking up their posts, newly registered nurses were only required to read the Trust's discharge planning policy. Beyond this, education relied upon the good will and time afforded to them by ward-based nurses interested in discharge planning.

There is little point in formulating new government policy without a serious commitment to deliver the changes required in practice. The Department of Health (2004) produced 'Achieving timely "simple" discharge from hospital: A toolkit for the multidisciplinary team'. This provided the foundation for an action plan, with a particular focus on the following elements:

- Core discharge skills analysis to determine areas of training required
- Competency assessment
- Competency-based training and declaration of competence

At this time, UCE Birmingham had just succeeded in its application to become a Centre of Excellence for Teaching and Learning (CETL). The lecturer involved won a bid for funding to support this new initiative. An external facilitator was appointed to oversee and support the new project as part of the CETL process. In developing any new initiatives, it is always important to consider funding. Developing new materials can be expensive, particularly when they involve multimedia technology. A cost analysis should be done at the outset to assess the time and money required to carry out any such project.

Deciding who the course is for

Who is the course for?

The programme was designed as a module that could be accessed by nurses and other health professionals studying at UCE Birmingham. It was also suggested that the module should be made available as a stand-alone course that could be marketed to other people outside the immediate area.

Universities give credits for modules of study that can be used to make up a defined award, as follows:

- Certificate level   120 credits
- Diploma level   120 credits
- Degree level   120 credits

It was decided that this module would be worth 12 credits at degree level.

Deciding on the content of the course

Course content

When designing study programmes it is important to consider the outcomes that the learner needs to demonstrate. In 2006, the Higher Education Academy (www.heacademy.ac.uk) put forward

Educational support for discharge planning

some points for consideration when designing a programme of learning:

1. What do you want students to know?
2. What do you want students to learn?
3. How will you create a syllabus using textbooks, research papers and personal research?
4. How can you develop resources to support students' learning?
5. How can you assess the knowledge students have gained?

There are some supplementary questions that may also be useful. First, what do you want students to be able to do? They need to listen, read, observe, discuss and argue, think for themselves, work independently and solve problems.

Secondly, how will you know what they have learnt? Students have to provide evidence to show that they can do something.

Thirdly, what do students, employers, and professional and statutory bodies think you should be teaching?

Fourthly, what competencies exist in this area of practice?

Consideration was given to all the above questions when designing the programme in Birmingham. The overall aims of the course should clearly explain what the teacher plans to deliver to the students, and the learning outcomes should describe clearly what the students will be able to do after completing the course or study module.

Before designing the aims and outcomes of the course, it is important to set the scene with a rationale explaining why this module of study is important. This should include all the relevant legislation and government policy.

The aims of the module

Aims of the module

The module aims to give the student an understanding of the political, social and economic implications of effective discharge planning. In addition, the module aims to give the student an appreciation of the roles of the nurse/therapist in the discharge planning process. The module should also give practitioners the skills required to develop a systematic, sustainable programme of change leading towards the introduction of nurse/therapist discharge.

When drawing up aims, it is important to remember that they are evidence of the goals set by a teacher or curriculum group

Background and theory

(Reece & Walker 2004, p. 16). Module aims are fairly general and should describe the overall purpose of the course.

The learning outcomes of the module

Learning outcomes translate the module aims into smaller, more specific, measurable components. When designing learning outcomes, it is important to tailor them to the particular type of learning involved. For example, learning can take place in the psycho-motor, cognitive or affective domain. Bloom (1984) designed a taxonomy of learning that allows for learning in each of these domains.

Some examples of specific learning outcomes for students are listed below.

1. Demonstrate an appreciation of the impact that government policy has on discharge planning
2. Demonstrate an understanding of the civil and legal frameworks that exist in relation to negligence, and how these impact on the roles of nurses and therapists who carry out the discharge of patients
3. Explore and apply strategies of change management for the introduction of nurse/therapist-led discharge planning
4. Critically appraise the role of the multi-professional team in ensuring that discharge planning is effective

Learning and teaching strategies used in the module

Learning and teaching strategies also need to be considered when designing new courses of study. We have already discussed some of the innovations that are impacting on education today. This module uses a blended style of learning, sometimes known as 'hybrid learning'. This combines delivery methods ranging from traditional classroom courses to self-paced learning on CD-ROM or the internet (Shank & Sitze 2004).

Information technology and use of the internet has been growing over the past 10 years. Introducing a range of blended learning approaches is an effective way to develop innovative learning materials. Courses should always utilise appropriate learning and teaching strategies. In the development of this module, the following strategies seemed appropriate:

- Problem-based learning
- Virtual learning environment
- Online learning

Educational support for discharge planning

At the development stage, it was important to involve the relevant departments within UCE Birmingham and the Hospital Foundation Trust. For example, part of the module was to be delivered using a virtual learning environment, which had to be designed using specific software available through one of the university departments. It is essential that all the relevant departments are included in the original plan, as it can delay proceedings if the required materials and resources are later found to be unavailable.

It was also decided that a range of short case studies would be presented online, and permission was sought from the hospital to contact health professionals who might be willing to contribute. It was thought that it would not be ethical to involve real patients in this exercise, as formal consent might be difficult to obtain and might prove too unsustainable. Staff were contacted and asked if they were interested in providing short video clips discussing their role. A mock ward round/case conference could also be set up. The following table shows ideas for developing short video clips that could be used within a virtual learning environment.

Ideas for video clips

Ideas for video clips

Job title	Subject for video clip
Intermediate care manager	Intermediate care services
	Single assessment process
Discharge liaison nurse	Discharge liaison roles and responsibilities
Social services manager	Coordination of social services
Continuing health manager	Reimbursement and recharging
Consultant nurse, Acute Medicine	Nurse-led discharge Estimating dates for discharge Protocol development Training needs analysis
Admissions and discharge manager	Coordination of bed management in a large NHS Trust

Some other subjects that could also be considered for short video clips, to be used in virtual learning environments, might include:

- A ward round
- A post-take ward round
- A multidisciplinary team meeting
- A bed management meeting
- An emergency assessment area
- A patient who has been discharged (not a real patient)

Background and theory

However, before embarking on the lengthy and costly process of producing this type of training material, it is worth clarifying a few questions, as suggested by Rowntree (1999):

- Who is expecting what of you?
- What resources can you call on in your project?
- How will you schedule your time?
- What media are available?
- If using video, have you got editing support?

Perhaps the most useful question to ask is: 'What is the simplest/cheapest medium or mix of media that will satisfactorily (even if not perfectly) meet our learners' needs?' (Rowntree 1999, p. 65).

There are several other questions to be considered when designing online materials. First, as we have seen, it is essential to decide on the right aims and learning outcomes at the planning stage. Learner support also needs to be taken into account, and how this support will be accessed. For example, there may already be materials available that could support the new module.

Scripts will need to be developed for video clips, and the sequence of ideas to be presented will need to be worked out. Support may also be needed from graphics and information technology experts.

The module that we designed in Birmingham was supported by the Centre for Teaching and Learning (CETL), which provided assistance in all of the above areas. The module material also included problem-based learning. This was designed using case studies that highlighted both the positive and negative aspects of patient discharge. Learners were expected to engage online with a support group to identify solutions and ways of improving discharge planning.

The module material also had to meet the requirements of the Special Educational Needs and Disability Act (2001), as it is important that equality and diversity are considered at all levels. Most universities have special departments set up to make sure that these requirements are met in any new material produced. This legislation is intended to widen participation in education and make education inclusive rather than exclusive.

The learning assessment strategy also needs to be clearly explained. For this particular module, there was a two-part assessment, with each part carrying 50 per cent of the total marks.

Educational support for discharge planning

The two parts were:

1. Completion of a reflective analysis of the discharge or transfer of a patient from hospital to home or other care setting (2,000 words)
2. Completion of a range of online tasks relevant to discharge planning (1,000 words)

The learning assessment strategy should test what learning has taken place and how this can be embedded in practice.

Mode of delivering the module

Delivering the module

It is envisaged that the module would be delivered in four main ways:

1. An induction day to introduce the learning materials and give students support in developing information technology skills
2. Online learning time in which activities would be continuously assessed as components of the module
3. Tutorial support to ensure that students are progressing with online material, producing a platform for reflective skills
4. An evaluation day to consolidate ongoing learning and evaluate the assessment strategy

The module would be delivered over a period of months, possibly as part of a formal academic semester or year. Some students might not choose to access the formal assessment but just wish to carry out the learning as an informal development exercise. Academic credits can only be awarded to students who have successfully achieved a pass grade in all aspects of the assessment strategy. Awarding universities usually have a formal process for awarding academic credits. Students who wish to have their credits formally acknowledged would usually have to register with the awarding university.

What are the essential elements in developing a successful training course?

Essential elements

Going back to the planning stage, it is advisable to check that clear instructions are given on how to access materials. Without clear instructions, students who are not proficient in information technology may soon become disheartened and de-motivated.

Background and theory

Innovative online and virtual materials should therefore be well planned and produced to a very high standard.

It may also be very helpful to pilot the course, using a few volunteers as students, before publishing it for the wider community. Rowntree (1999) suggests that piloting may be the most crucial task in the whole project, following the pattern:

- Write it
- Try it out
- Improve it

Feedback from pilot stages is essential to ensure that your final version is both credible and marketable. This feedback should include critical commenting and continuous monitoring. Most online and virtual learning environments incorporate ways of recording how many learners have utilised the resource, so immediate feedback is usually available.

Factors that need to be considered when designing online learning materials include:

- Type of learner
- Encouragement of self-directed ability
- Staff access to computers via libraries and on wards
- Mandatory training for any new staff as part of induction programme
- Most up-to-date media system for computer use

Evaluation

In evaluating a module, it may be useful to consider a stakeholder analysis. This looks at how the programme has impacted upon all the interested parties. A typical stakeholder analysis is shown below.

Stakeholder analysis for evaluation of module

Stakeholder analysis

Interested party/parties	Impact
Any co-authors	
Colleagues or managers	
Learners' online managers	
Pilot learners and tutors	
Foundation Trust colleagues	
Consultants	
Accrediting bodies	
Others	
Patients and carers	

Educational support for discharge planning

The technology also has to be cost-effective, and production costs have to be clearly worked out. Most universities have a set price for modules (i.e. amount paid per student taking the module). This can range from as little as £100 to as much as £1,000, depending on the level and mode of delivery. The cost of updating information, which can quickly become outdated in the health service arena, also needs to be taken into account.

The long-term delivery platform should also be considered. Educational and practice areas could gain invaluable experience in delivering online courses. This can lead to new developments, with mobile phones, for example, being used as a means of providing learning materials for students.

Marketing the course is another important element. For instance, events such as conferences and networking meetings can provide valuable opportunities to market innovative education packages.

Course material should always be appraised in an immediate and constructive way but simple oversights may prevent this. For example, students may not be able to access existing materials because their computers do not have the right software.

Other factors

Other factors to be considered when developing learning materials have been outlined by Lewis and Allan (2005), as follows:

- **Overall design principles** such as the use of audio and video technology
- **Methods and techniques**, which could include the use of formative and summative assessment tools
- **Individual learning styles**, which should be considered to ensure that a range of students could engage with the material
- **Development of knowledge**, which could be tested during and at the end of any period of learning
- **Changes in professional practice**, which could be demonstrated through the use of competencies that have to be achieved as part of the material
- **Impact on the organisation**, including the development of staff utilising information technology as part of their everyday work
- **Impact on the virtual learning organisation**, such as encouraging the interactive use of the internet and the sharing of information and best practice.

Training time for all students and staff should be built into their overall schedules. And, as previously mentioned, the cost of this should be included in the overall costs of delivering the module.

Conclusion

Developing learning materials for effective discharge planning is an exciting initiative. The particular module discussed in this chapter was produced for practitioners who had already gained an initial qualification in their own area of practice (such as nursing, physiotherapy, occupational therapy or social work). The module aims to help members of the multidisciplinary team assess their own level of knowledge and skill in the discharge planning process. It should help to identify training needs and it could be studied alone or as part of a more formal programme of learning such as a diploma or degree or higher award such as a master's degree or doctorate.

The components of the module and the interactive material could be adapted for use by other staff such as healthcare assistants and students from allied healthcare professions. Newly qualified staff could study this module as part of a development programme or supervisory programme. Expert practitioners and consultants could also use the material as a reflective aid to ensure that they are delivering best practice in discharge planning.

Final tips for success in developing training programmes include:
- Taking a collaborative approach to developing new material
- Following professional practice guidelines
- Utilising expertise to develop interactive materials
- Ensuring that learners are supported

Educational support for discharge planning

References

Bloom, B.S.(1984). *Taxonomy of educational objectives*. Boston: Pearson Education.

Department of Health (2004). 'Achieving timely "simple" discharge from Hospital: A toolkit for the multidisciplinary team'. London: The Stationery Office.

Department for Education and Skills (2004). 'The Future of Higher Education'. London: The Stationery Office.

Harris, A. (1997). *Needs to Know: A guide to needs assessment for Primary Care Nurses*. Edinburgh: Churchill Livingstone.

Health Commission (2004). 'Patient Survey Report'. London: Health Commission.

Health Professions Council (2005). 'Continuing Professional Development: Key Decisions'. London: Health Professions Council.

Higher Education Academy (2006). 'Some ways of designing a course page'. (www.heacademy.ac.uk/1555.htm)

Higher Education Funding Council (2004). 'Learning and Teaching: Teaching Initiatives: Centres for Excellence in Teaching and Learning'. (www.hefce.ac.uk/learning/tinits/cetl/)

Howell Major, C. & Savin-Baden, M. (2004). *Foundations of problem-based learning*. Society for Research into Higher Education and the Open University. Berkshire: Open University Press.

Jisc infonet (2006). Infokit. Analytical Tools and Templates. (www.jiscinfonet.ac.uk)

Lewis, D. & Allan, B. (2005). *Virtual Learning Communities: a guide for practitioners*. The Society for Research into Higher Education. Berkshire: Open University Press.

Nursing and Midwifery Council (2004). *The PREP Handbook*. London: Nursing and Midwifery Council.

Quality Assurance Agency for Higher Education (2001). The Quality Assurance Agency for Higher Education: an introduction. (www.qaa.ac.uk)

Reece, I. & Walker, S. (2003). *Teaching, Training and Learning: A Practical Guide Incorporating FENTO Standards* (5th edn.) Hampshire: Dance Books Ltd.

Rowntree, D. (1994). *Preparing Materials for Open, Distance and Flexible Learning*. London: Kogan Page.

Background and theory

SENDA (2001). The Special Educational Needs and Disability Act 2001. London: The Stationery Office.

Shank, P. & Sitze, A. (2004). *Making Sense of Online Learning: A Guide for Beginners and the Truly Skeptical.* San Francisco: Pfeiffer Wiley.

Weller, M. (2002). *Delivering Learning on the Net: The Why, What and How of Online Education.* London: Routledge Farmer

Chapter 4

Competency and role development

Denise Price and Lyn Garbarino

This chapter discusses the issues involved in developing, maintaining and assessing discharge competence. The Royal College of Nursing Core Career and Competence Framework (Royal College of Nursing 2006) and discharge planning competencies are used to demonstrate the practical application of these skills. An overview of the Knowledge and Skills Framework (KSF) is provided to enable the reader to see the chapter as a practical guide in the workplace context, exploring the impact of both discharge competencies and the KSF in practice.

An overview of competencies

Overview of competencies

Competence was described by the United Kingdom Central Council (UKCC) in 1999, in relation to practice, as 'the skills and ability to practise safely and effectively without the need for direct supervision' (UKCC 1999). This definition was embraced by the 'NHS Plan' (2000); and other recent government initiatives have focused firmly on the need to develop a competent workforce. This approach gathered momentum during 2004, when competence was described in broader terms by the Nursing and Midwifery Council, which stated: 'to practise competently, you must possess the knowledge, skills and abilities required for lawful, safe and effective practice without direct supervision' (NMC 2004).

Competencies form a framework that clearly demonstrates the skills required to undertake any particular part of a practitioner's role, and they are a valuable tool for career planning (McAleer *et al.*

Background and theory

1997, Skills for Health 2004, Royal College of Nursing 2005). They create transparency about what is collectively required in terms of knowledge and skills. They also illustrate the standard expected at assessment, and ensure that knowledge is evidence-based and reflected in practice. Clinical and professional development within nursing depends on the accumulation of clinical skills of differing degrees of complexity.

Roach (1992) describes competence as 'the state of having the knowledge, judgement, skills, energy, experience and motivation required to respond adequately to the demands of one's professional responsibilities'. And Benner (1984) proposed that in the acquisition and development of a skill, a student passes through five levels of competence: novice, advanced beginner, competent, proficient and expert. Clearly, there is no shortage of people ready to define competence and its usefulness in taking the nursing profession forward to new and more advanced roles.

As far as the education and ongoing professional development of nurses are concerned, there is a definite move towards incorporating work-based and lifelong learning to support individuals in achieving and maintaining their professional competence (Milligan 1998). The Project 2000 curriculum shifted away from a purely skills- or competency-based approach to professional development, which included a degree or diploma level of academic preparation. In doing so, it moved learning further away from the workplace (McCormack & Kenefic 1991, Watkins 2000). Competencies, however, facilitate work-based learning within the context of the practitioner's own area of practice. This allows practitioners to gain insights and knowledge that support their own individual practice (Flanagan et al. 2000).

Ashworth and Sexton (1990) describe how a purely competency-based approach can reduce nursing to mechanistic tasks and devalue more advanced roles. It would be a backward step for nursing training to focus solely upon the acquisition of behavioural and motor skills. New roles require a balance of theory and practical experience. This combination enables the practitioner to incorporate the critical and analytical skills developed through more formal education routes, including an outcome-based competency approach to learning.

Competency and role development

Which comes first – competence or the new role?

New roles are often developed at times when healthcare organisations are extending or advancing nursing responsibilities or changing skill mix structures within clinical areas. The first step in creating a new or redesigned role is usually to draw up a job description and person specification. Yet the starting point should really be the competencies required to deliver effective outcome-based clinical care (Skills for Health 2004).

As competencies are used to describe and analyse a role in detail, they make a good basis for developing job specifications, redesigning roles and formulating recruitment strategies (Skills for Health 2004). This means that the specific required competencies remain central to the role's initial and ongoing development. A task-orientated approach to nursing moves practice away from the principles of holistic care. In contrast, contextualising care, by respecting the individual patient's values and beliefs, prevents nursing from becoming purely mechanistic (McAleer & Hamill 1997, Watkins 2000).

Watkins (2000) describes how work-based competencies should ensure that developing nursing skills in line with evidence from practice becomes the norm. New roles need to be developed by considering the competencies required to achieve desired patient outcomes. The skills of professionals can then be more effectively matched with the needs of the patient (Flanagan *et al.* 2000).

A competence framework

Competence framework

A competence framework often contains a number of statements defining what individuals or teams need to know and should be able to do, in order to deliver a service (Skills for Health 2004, Davis *et al.* 2003). A particular competency also clearly demonstrates the level of knowledge, values, attitudes and skills required for that element of practice (Flanagan *et al.* 2000).

The framework can be constructed around the competencies required by an individual practitioner. Alternatively, a framework may include a much broader set of competencies required by the wider multi-professional team, in order to deliver the whole service or support the patient pathway. A competency-based approach can

Background and theory

also be used to highlight gaps and duplications in service between professional groups and individuals, helping to identify new ways of working and new or redesigned roles. This provides an effective way of developing services across organisational or professional boundaries. Using this approach, skills and competencies are aligned to the relevant people working within the service, irrespective of which part of the organisation they come from.

Assessing competence

Assessing competence

Evaluating and assessing clinical nursing competence is an important part of professional development (Lee-Hsieh *et al.* 2003). Indeed, Neary (2000) and Watkins (2000) have shown that nurses definitely appreciate the assessment of their clinical competence. They see this evaluation as a valuable step in developing both individual practice and a level of competence across a whole team or ward environment.

Assessment of nurses clearly needs to focus on performance over a period of time in the clinical area, rather than simply looking at behavioural changes observed during a one-off assessment. Work-based learning allows for an assessment over time, taking into account the value of learning within the clinical workplace, and acknowledging how nurses carry out their actual work (Hinchliff 2000, Parish 2001). This requires the support of trained assessors who are objective and therefore able to give feedback that encourages and supports personal development and safe practice (While 1994).

The following table lists the advantages and disadvantages of a number of assessment methods and is intended to provide a quick reference tool for assessment planning (Lee-Hsieh *et al.* 2003, Flanagan *et al.* 2000, Davis *et al.* 2003, Girot 2000, Scholes *et al.* 2004, Watkins 2000).

Assessment of competence depends on the ability to demonstrate and apply existing knowledge and skills, and this applies both to competence of practice and to 'The NHS Knowledge and Skills Framework' (KSF). The starting point for assessment should be a comparison of prior learning (as demonstrated by the nurse) against local discharge planning competencies or those described later in this chapter.

Assessment methods

The advantages and disadvantages of different assessment methods		
Assessment type	Advantages	Disadvantages
Self-evaluation	Good as a pre-test of own knowledge and skills.	Often score higher when evaluating self.
Peer/mentor evaluations	Assessment can be a continuous process, not a one-off activity.	Need to observe and monitor closely to gain a true reflection of competence. Peers and/or mentors also need training and/or support.
Testing (verbal and/or written)	Predetermined criteria required.	Could be seen as time-consuming and onerous. Allows for a more academic type of examination, with pass or fail criteria.
Work-based learning (learning sets, clinical seminars, practice-based projects and assessment, reflective diaries, skills inventories, learning contracts)	Brings together self-knowledge, formal knowledge and expertise at work. Maximises the opportunities for learning and professional development. Supports lifelong learning that is responsive to change. Supports a focused approach to development needs.	The learner must want to learn in the workplace. The work environment must be suitably prepared and conducive to learning. The learning must be within the learner's capabilities.
Personal portfolio	Provides evidence of achievement of specific competencies, transferable skills and learning. Supports role and career transition and academic development. Supports reflective practice.	Requires time and patience to develop effectively. Training required in effective portfolio development. Collects a range of practice-based evidence and dialogue. Creates an inventory of transferable skills.

The type of evidence that demonstrates prior learning and experience of discharge planning can be agreed at local level. This may range from case studies to evidence of research or literature reviews, observation of current discharge practice followed by a reflective piece, and/or observation of the individual's own discharge practice, with signed testimonials. Whichever type of evidence is used, it is always vital to have a clear and consistent process for teaching, assessing and maintaining competence, and this approach needs to be standardised across an organisation or care pathway. As discharge can involve several professional groups and agencies, evidence of the nurse's competence should only reflect the part of the discharge planning process for which that nurse is responsible.

The table on p. 61 demonstrates the advantages and disadvantages of a number of different assessment approaches. The assessment method selected should be the one best suited to the learning style of the individual nurse, as this will achieve optimum results for both the individual and the organisation.

Timescales for achieving competence will vary according to the nurse's prior learning and experience. Gaining competence over a protracted period of time (stretching from months into years) devalues the assessment process and the actual worth of competency frameworks themselves. As discharge planning is an essential part of the nursing role, gaining competence should be demonstrated within a short timescale (either weeks or months), and this should be agreed at the beginning between the nurse and assessor.

Assessment of competence places an increased burden on already overstretched assessors in practice, so a pragmatic approach may be required when it comes to deciding who 'signs off' the competence itself. At the very least, this responsibility should be taken by a nurse or allied health professional with a different or higher level of expertise from the nurse being assessed, and the assessor should be recognised locally as undertaking this role. This means that every nurse with the appropriate level of experience can potentially become an assessor of competence.

Reviewing competence

Reviewing competence

Competencies need to be regularly reviewed in the light of changing clinical practice and patient need. As competencies combine relevant theory and practice, they provide a tool for testing both these elements within clinical practice (Milligan 1998). In maintaining the safe use of any competency, the ability to rehearse and use the relevant skills in an environment that promotes learning is crucial (Watkins 2000, NMC 2004).

Organisations often focus on the short-term acquisition of skills at the expense of lifelong learning (Campbell 2004). However, through the review and monitoring process (which is integral to the development of competencies), explicit links can be made between current clinical practice, annual appraisal, self-reflection and lifelong learning (Davis *et al.* 2003). 'The NHS Knowledge and Skills Framework' (KSF) is designed to identify how the knowledge and skills required by individuals are actually applied in practice. The KSF also provides a fair and objective framework on which to base the review and development of individuals (DoH 2004).

A closer look at the Knowledge and Skills Framework

Knowledge and Skills Framework

The Department of Health describes the KSF as 'a broad generic framework that focuses on the application of knowledge and skills but does not describe the exact knowledge and skills that individuals need to develop. More specific standards or competencies will achieve this along with the outcomes of learning programmes' (DoH 2004, p. 5).

The KSF is made up of 30 dimensions, each broadly identifying functions required to provide a quality service to the patient. There are six core dimensions:

1. Communication
2. Personal and people development
3. Health, safety and security
4. Service improvement
5. Quality
6. Equality and diversity

The remaining 24 dimensions are specific, grouped into four themes and applied to specific NHS roles:

1. Health and well-being
2. Estates and facilities
3. Information and knowledge
4. General

Each dimension has four levels, and each level has one or more indicators that describe how knowledge and skills need to be applied at that level.

In summary, the KSF has four main aims, listed below:

1. To facilitate the development of services, through investing in the development of all staff members, so that they can better meet the needs of users

Background and theory

2. To support the effective learning and development of individuals and teams
3. To support the development of individuals in their posts, so that they are effective at work
4. To promote equality and diversity of all staff, using the framework for learning and development

The Knowledge and Skills Framework (KSF) provides a new impetus and incentive to use competencies as the basis for role development. It also encourages a truly patient-focused approach to designing new roles. Skills for Health (the new Skills Council for Health) has created hundreds of competencies. These competencies all take the following questions as their starting points (*Health Service Journal* 2004, p. 1):

- What does the service need to deliver?
- What does the workforce need to look like, in terms of competencies and skills?
- What is the existing knowledge base?

Embedding competencies and the KSF within work-based learning

Embedding competencies

If competencies and the KSF are to have a positive impact on practice and lead to improvements in patient care and services, their outcomes must be made explicit to individual nurses. Campbell (2004) and the Department of Health (2003) described how a key element of clinical governance is ensuring that health professionals get the education, training, skills and competencies they need to deliver necessary care to patients.

During the annual appraisal process, the competencies and KSF will form a robust framework from which the development needs of an individual can be clearly identified. By linking the assessment of competence with the KSF, evidence can be provided that supports the attainment of the competence itself and also includes examples of application of the specific dimension required for KSF. The combined framework enables a detailed personal development plan to be agreed, linked to appropriate learning and development (DoH 2004). The diagram below demonstrates the benefits of a combined competency and KSF framework, for the patient, for the individual nurse and for the employer.

Competency and role development

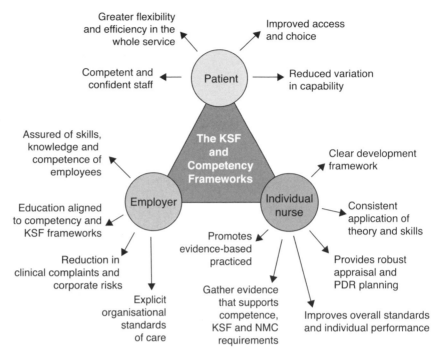

The benefits of a combined KSF and competency framework

The Royal College of Nursing Core Career and Competency Framework

The Royal College of Nursing (RCN) Framework enables practitioners to track their competence development as they progress through the career levels, applying it to the specialist area of practice in which they work. It shows how the different dimensions and levels within the KSF might be appropriate at different career stages in nursing. The NHS KSF (2004) has been used as the basis for the RCN 'Core Career and Competency Framework'.

The RCN Framework is linked to earlier work on competencies, undertaken by the RCN, to ensure that the nurse is meeting the expected levels for career progression, according to the Agenda for Change (AfC). AfC is the system of pay put in place in 2004 for most NHS-employed staff, with the exception of doctors. It also identifies the knowledge and skills that need to be applied to specific practice areas. Thus, through using the RCN Framework, nurses will be able to, for example, demonstrate evidence of competence at four different levels in general and specialist areas of nursing. They will also be able to show readiness to progress to the next career level, using professional accreditation tools.

Career and competency framework

Background and theory

The documents are lengthy but it should be noted that not all dimensions of the KSF identified at each level of career progression are needed to attain competence at that level. The dimensions chosen should be based on the job description, not the person. They will therefore vary according to the context in which the nurse works. All six core dimensions of the KSF (described on p. 63) need to be attained at each level of career progression. However, it is recommended that about four other dimensions are also chosen, depending upon the job held by the nurse. The KSF levels of attainment will also vary according to the job.

Competence levels

The RCN competence levels are identified as follows:

- **Competent nurse:** a newly qualified nurse gaining experience in a practice area, or a nurse who transfers from one area of practice to another where different specialist skills are required
- **Experienced nurse:** a nurse with some experience of caring for patients within a specific client group, who now mentors other nurses, and who is working to protocols and guidelines and making clinical decisions
- **Senior practitioner:** a nurse who is leading a team of more junior staff or undertaking a specialist role
- **Consultant nurse:** an expert nurse with parallel expertise in education, research and consultancy in practice

These levels are based on the career trajectory, defined by the Department of Health (DoH 1999), which suggests that competence is cumulative. Senior practitioners would be expected to achieve their own level of competency statements, in addition to those of the competent and experienced levels. It is envisaged that the Nursing and Midwifery Council (NMC) domains and competencies for advanced nurse practitioners will match the senior practitioner level, as described in the RCN 'Core Career and Competency Framework'. Therefore a nurse working as an advanced nurse practitioner in discharge planning should be working to the senior practitioner framework and applying that to their practice.

Recent developments have seen the linking of a number of Skills for Health (SfH) competencies to the RCN 'Core Career and Competency Framework'. These have been drawn from a large portfolio of competencies based on National Occupational Standards and National Workforce Competencies. SfH identify competencies required by those providing and delivering care in various contexts. Thus, these competencies are not profession-specific but are required by those involved in care across pathways.

The collaboration between Skills for Health and the RCN provides a tried and tested competency framework, with building blocks that are either nurse- or profession-specific. Developing these within the context of discharge planning would require experienced practitioners to identify exactly what skills are needed to be able to discharge patients effectively.

RCN framework

KSF Dimension: Core 1. COMMUNICATION Level: 3 Develop and maintain communication with people about difficult matters and/or in difficult situations		
Indicators	Areas of application to nursing practice with examples (core)	Skills for Health – National Workforce Competencies/National Occupational Standards
a) Identifies the range of people likely to be involved in the communication, and any potential communication differences and relevant contextual factors	a) Communicates effectively and appropriately with: • patients, those important to patients, users • the nursing team • the interdisciplinary team (i.e. social workers, doctors, bed managers, modern matrons, allied health professionals, administrative staff, housekeeping staff) • other healthcare professionals	HSC31 Promote communication for and about individuals
b) Communicates with people in a form and manner that: • is consistent with their level of understanding, culture, background and preferred ways of communicating • is appropriate to the purpose of the communication and the context in which it is taking place • encourages the effective participation of all involved	b) Communicates with patients/users/others: • in an appropriate person-centred manner consistent with their level of understanding, culture and background, preferred ways of communicating and needs (i.e. is empathetic to patients/users/others) • develops a good rapport with patients/users/others • acts as an advocate for the patients/clients/carers according to their wishes • enables participation	HSC31 Promote communication for and about individuals

The table above shows an extract from the RCN Framework at Competent Level. The first column is the KSF Core Dimension 1

(Communication), at Level 3. The second column is application to practice from a generic perspective. The third column is Skills for Health competencies that align to this domain. The full RCN document is available online at www.rcn.org.uk and details of the Skills for Health competencies are available on www.skillsforhealth.org.uk.

The RCN 'Core Career and Competency Framework' has taken three years to develop, requiring intense collaboration both internally within the RCN and externally. The RCN Professional Forums have already undertaken a considerable amount of work. Indeed the RCN Framework has provided the basis for several specialist frameworks. The specialist frameworks are also available on the RCN website (e.g. Occupational Health, Outpatients, Dermatology, Trauma and Orthopaedics) and have provided a focus for nurses already working within these specialist areas. At this stage, there is no specific RCN framework for discharge planning but one could be built very quickly using the models that have already been developed, combined with input from experts from the field.

Relating competencies to discharge planning

Relating competencies to planning

In the current ever-changing healthcare climate, practitioners lack the time and resources to undertake extra work. It therefore makes sense to utilise the competency frameworks that have already been developed. In cases where competency models are tried, tested and recommended, these can easily be applied to practice. For example, one way forward would be to adopt the generic components of the RCN Framework and combine them with a specialist discharge planning framework.

In fact, a discharge planning model has already been developed, with full expert nursing and multi-professional support. This is the matrix of training competencies for timely discharge, presented in the Department of Health document (2004), 'Achieving timely "simple" discharge from hospital'. This framework is designed for any member of the multidisciplinary team to use, whether they are deemed to be at novice, experienced or expert level.

The tables on pages 70 and 71 provide an illustration of the matrix of training competencies for timely discharge.

Competency and role development

The core knowledge and skills for professionals with discharge planning responsibility are listed below:

- Working within a multidisciplinary team
- Estimating the expected date of discharge
- Developing, implementing and reviewing the clinical management plan
- Making referrals
- Interpreting test results and investigations

The specific discharge planning competencies required can be adjusted to fit whichever environment the discharge takes place in. For example, the patient may be discharged to a variety of settings, such as their own home, intermediate care, outreach settings or longer-term care such as a nursing home or residential home.

Discharge practice does not remain static. Indeed, one discharge liaison nurse commented that this was the first time that 'anyone had ever bothered to think about discharge practice as more than an assumed nursing skill'. The competencies were seen as raising the status of those in discharge planning roles and affording specialist skills to those working in a vastly undervalued area of clinical practice.

Within each level, the practitioner is expected to assess themselves and identify whether they are competent, partially competent, or have not yet had the necessary experience that underpins the knowledge and the skill to be a competent discharge planner. This framework allows for self-assessment and peer review of the range of knowledge and skills required. It can be included as part of a personal development plan to ensure that any further training required is undertaken. Thus, the need to provide a safe, effective service and to achieve the expected dimensions in the KSF are both addressed in a single plan.

Conclusion

The 'NHS Plan' (DoH 2000) and the pay reforms identified in Agenda for Change focus on the need to develop a competent workforce. By using the tools already developed or adapting them to meet the local context, practitioners can avoid having to re-invent the wheel. They can also demonstrate that effective care is being provided as well as meeting their personal agendas and

Background and theory

	Multidisciplinary team (MDT) working	Estimating expected date of discharge (EDD)	Development, implementation and review of clinical management plan (CMP)
Advanced Practitioners (Expert) Able to make decisions independently	Able to: ● Lead a team effectively ● Demonstrate collaborative working and has trust of senior colleagues ● Communicate effectively with team/other HCP/patients and carers ● Develop/implement clinical management plan ● Identify and achieve shared goals	Able to: ● Undertake full assessment of the patient including physical, physiological, social and functional ● Demonstrate excellent knowledge of the clinical condition and the investigations/interventions required ● Estimate the length of stay needed to complete treatment to a level where the patient is clinically fit for discharge ● Review and revise EDD based on further assessment/data	Able to: ● Develop clinical management plan based on full assessment ● Implement and review CMP developed by another member of MDT ● Review patient progress and adjust the plan in response to assessment and test results ● Identify EDD within the plan ● Demonstrate ability to make effective discharge decisions
Practitioners (Experienced) (Completed foundation year) Able to present all information needed for decision making but require support in making decisions	Able to: ● Demonstrate good understanding of individual roles within MDT and their contribution to discharge ● Communicates effectively with members of MDT/patients/carers ● Anticipates information needed by MDT in order to make decisions ● Demonstrates high level of knowledge of discharge process	Able to: ● Undertake partial assessment of the patient including physical, physiological, social and functional ● Use protocols/guidelines/ICPs to support planning and implementation of care ● Prompt MDT to estimate EDD and document in patient record ● Prompt review of EDD based on assessment of patient	Able to: ● Implement aspects of the CMP and coordinate care around the patient ● Assess the patient (clinical condition specific) for discharge, using criteria or protocols developed by MDT ● Identify when patient's condition has deteriorated and patient is no longer suitable for discharge
Newly Qualified Practitioners (Novice) (During foundation year) Able to demonstrate an understanding of discharge process	Able to: ● Demonstrate an awareness of individual roles within MDT ● Understand the importance of effective and timely communication	Able to: ● Carry out basic components of assessment ● Follow instructions and to report any variances to team leaders ● Demonstrate awareness of impotance in discharge model	Able to: ● Demonstrate understanding of elements of CMP ● Implement aspects of the plan under supervision ● Demonstrate understanding of importance of effective documentation and communication

	Making referrals	Interpretation of test results and investigations	Patient decides to self discharge against healthcare professional advice
Advanced Practitioners (Expert) Able to make decisions independently	Able to: ● Demonstrate excellent ability to identify when a referral is needed ● Initiate referral to other members of MDT ● Follow up actions and results from referrals ● Coordinate and run MDT review of patient ● Use outcome of MDT review to adopt CMP and EDD	Able to: ● Refer and interpret test results ● Adjust CMP in response to the results of tests and investigations ● Identify when future discussion and review by medical colleagues and other members of MDT ● Take responsibility for discharge decision based on clinical assessment and best results	Able to: ● Attempt to persuade patient to remain in hospital if this is in the clinical interest of the patient ● Explain the risks and potential consequences of self discharge to the patient and carers ● Rapidly coordinate care package if accepted by the patient ● Document events accurately within patient record ● Communicate with GP, including discharge letter
Practitioners (Experienced) (Completed foundation year) Able to present all information needed for decision making but require support in making decisions	Able to: ● Recognise when referral to MDT may be needed ● Make referrals based on guidance from others ● Coordinate actions and results from referrals ● Demonstrate understanding of MDT review and implications for CMP and EDD	Able to: ● Proactively chase test results ● Understand the significance of test results ● Communicate abnormal test results effectively and in a timely manner to appropriate member of MDT	Able to: ● Explore reasons for self discharge ● Inform patient's consultant or senior medical team of patient's intention ● Ensure all relevant documentation is completed
Newly Qualified Practitioners (Novice) (During foundation year) Able to demonstrate an understanding of discharge process	Able to: ● Follow instructions and plans developed by other members of MDT ● Document when referrals have been made in patient record	Able to: ● Accurately record and document test results ● Demonstrate an awareness of normal and abnormal test results	Able to: ● Demonstrate awareness of the risks and potential consequences of self discharge for patient ● Demonstrate awareness of the policy and procedures/documentation required

addressing the KSF. However, this presents a challenge for many nurses. There is a perception that competency frameworks are a means of 'policing' the service!

There is therefore a need to embed competence development into the healthcare culture, so that it becomes the norm rather than an optional extra. This will only happen when the importance of competence development and the value of a competent workforce are recognised. Staff members need to be engaged in developing the frameworks and feel ownership of the work. Ideally, competence needs to be linked to the patient pathway so that all aspects of care along the pathway are underpinned by the knowledge and skills needed to provide that care.

Discharge competencies could be embraced by all the professionals included in the multidisciplinary team and help define goals for the patient along the pathway. They can also be linked to competence frameworks already developed by other professionals to avoid repetition. This means breaking down barriers and recognising that individuals cannot work in isolation. It is also a way of sharing responsibility in terms of who assesses competence levels.

When the KSF is used to full advantage and personal development plans are systematically linked to appraisals this change may well become evident.

In conclusion, if the KSF is not taken on board and used as a positive tool to help develop a safe, effective healthcare service then 'competence' may turn out to be another briefly fashionable term that is soon forgotten.

References

Avon, Gloucestershire and Wiltshire WDC (2004). 'Introduction to role redesign'. Wiltshire: AGW Strategic Health Authority.

Ashworth, P.D. & Saxton, J. (1990). 'On competence'. *Journal of Further and Higher Education*, 14, 3–25.

Benner, P.E. (1984). *From Novice to Expert: Excellence and Power in Clinical Nursing Practice*. California: Addison Wesley Publishing Company.

Campbell, S. (2004). 'Continuing Professional Development: What do we need?' *Nursing Management*, 10 (10), 27–31.

Davis, N. & Bheenuck, S. (2003). 'A professional development pathways scheme'. *Nursing Standard*, 17 (48), 40–43.

Department of Health (2000). 'The NHS Plan: A plan for investment, a plan for reform'. London: The Stationery Office.

Department of Health (2003). 'Discharge from hospital: Pathway, process and practice'. London: The Stationery Office.

Department of Health (2004). 'The NHS Knowledge and Skills Framework (NHS KSF) and the Development Review process'. London: The Stationery Office.

Department of Health (2004). 'Achieving timely "simple" discharge from hospital: A toolkit for the multidisciplinary team'. London: The Stationery Office.

Department of Health (2004). 'Agenda for Change'. London: The Stationery Office.

Eraut, M. (1998). 'Concepts of competence'. *Journal of Interprofessional Care*, 12 (2), 127–139.

Flanagan, J., Baldwin, S. & Clarke, D. (2000). 'Work-based learning as a means of developing and assessing nursing competence'. *Journal of Clinical Nursing*, 9, 360–368.

Girot, E.A. (2000). 'Assessment of graduates and diplomats in practice in the UK – are we measuring the same level of competence?' *Journal of Clinical Nursing*, 9, 330–337.

Health Service Journal (2004). 'The future of skills'. An HSJ supplement, 1–9.

Hinchliff, S. (2000). 'Accreditation'. *Nursing Standard*, 15 (3), 33–34.

James, C. (1995). 'Professional education – who learns what?' *Nurse Education Today*, 15, 161–163.

Background and theory

Lee-Hsieh, J., Kao, C., Kuo, C. & Tseng, H. (2003). 'Clinical Nursing Competence of RN-to-BSN Students in a Nursing Concept Based Curriculum'. *Taiwan Journal of Nursing Education*, 42 (12), 536–546.

McAleer, J. & Hamill, C. (1997). 'The Assessment of Higher Order Competence Development in Nurse Education: Executive Summary'.
Belfast: University of Ulster.

McCormack, B. & Kenefic, D. (1991). *Learning on the Job*.
London: Souvenir Press.

Milligan, F. (1998). 'Defining and assessing competence: the distraction of outcomes and the importance of educational process'. *Nurse Education Today*, 18, 273–280.

Neary, M. (2000). 'Responsive assessment: Assessing student nurses' clinical competence'. *Nurse Education Today*, 21 (1), 3–17.

Nursing and Midwifery Council (2004). 'The NMC code of professional conduct: standards for conduct, performance and ethics'. London: NMC.

Parish, C. (2001). 'Learn while you work'. *Nursing Standard*, 16 (2), 16–17.

Royal College of Nursing (2005). 'Competencies: an integrated career and competency framework for dermatology nursing'. London: RCN.

Royal College of Nursing (2006). 'Core Career and Competency Framework'.
London: RCN. (www.rcn.org.uk/resources/corecompetences/)

Scholes, J., Webb, C., Gray, M., Endacott, R., Miller, C., Jasper, M. & Mcmullan, M. (2004). 'Making portfolios work in practice'. *Journal of Advanced Nursing*, 46 (6), 595–603.

Skills for Health (2004). 'Older People's National Workforce Competence Framework Guide'. Bristol: Skills for Health.

United Kingdom Central Council (1999). 'Fitness for Practice: the UKCC Commission for Nursing and Midwifery Education'. London: UKCC.

Watkins, M.J. (2000). 'Competency for nursing practice'.
Journal of Clinical Nursing, 9, 338–346.

While, A. (1994). 'Competence versus performance: which is more important?'
Journal of Advanced Nursing, 20, 525–531.

Section 2

Clinical practice considerations

Chapter 5

Maintaining strategic organisational momentum through senior nursing input

Alison Wells

This chapter discusses the role of nurses in maintaining strategic organisational momentum when improving discharge practice. Government policy both informs and reflects this aspect of nursing, so it may be useful to begin by looking at policy developments over the last two decades.

The need to reduce the length of stay for patients (in order to increase bed occupancy in acute hospitals) has been on the political agenda for a number of years. In 1989 a Department of Health Circular (HC 89 5) requested that health authorities review their discharge procedures. The Patients' Charter (1991) contained standards outlining what patients could expect on discharge from hospital. Since then, there have been a number of publications and the government's expectations have become more explicit.

The Healthcare Commission has outlined three main principles relating to the discharge of patients. These are:
- To avoid hospitalisation wherever possible
- To keep people 'out of the care system wherever appropriate'
- To provide 'fair and prompt access to care'

The Healthcare Commission carries out an 'annual health check' across the healthcare economy. This is a framework of national targets and standards set out by the government to encourage healthcare improvements and help patients and the public make better-informed choices. The assessment is carried out across all NHS providers each year, with the first report due for publication in October 2006.

The annual health check includes a commitment from Trusts to reduce the number of delayed transfers of care. Managing the flow of patients has a clear impact on discharge practice. Trusts are expected to reduce length of patient stay and increase patient turnover, and more efficient discharge practice can help deliver these two goals.

The responsibility for improving the discharge process lies with the whole of the multidisciplinary team (DoH 2003, 2004b) but, inevitably, it will mainly fall upon nurses who have contact with patients 24 hours a day, 7 days a week. Additionally, Board-level nurses frequently have responsibility for allied health professionals within an organisation, so non-medical multidisciplinary working will also fall into their remit. This chapter focuses on the role of nurses in maintaining organisational momentum. However, the needs of different wards and departments should also be considered. In some of these settings, it may be more appropriate for leadership to be provided by other members of the multidisciplinary team (Pethybridge 2004).

Board-level nurses' responsibilities

Nurses' responsibility

For efficient, effective discharge to become part of everyday practice, the focus on discharge has to be absorbed into nursing culture in general. This means that nurses 'on the shop floor' need to be enthused. This also applies to junior doctors whose multifaceted responsibilities often mean that discharge planning may not be a high priority for them. Without a high level of motivation and collaboration between nurses, doctors and allied health professionals, it is impossible to have an impact on discharge practice.

Traditionally, nurses have believed that patients are better off in hospital and have worried about discharging them too early. This contradicts research, which shows that longer stays in hospital can result in deterioration in a patient's condition and an increase in mortality (Steel, Gertman *et al.* 2004, Clarke 2002). In addition, there is a cynicism regarding national targets because these targets are seen as being driven by financial pressures rather than patient needs (Drake, Bore *et al.* 2004). However, in relation to discharge, a shorter hospital stay will benefit most patients.

The method of implementing change is crucial for its sustainability. Evidence shows that change is most successful if it is locally owned. However, practitioners' enthusiasm, once gained, has to be channelled to ensure continuing action. This can only be achieved if there is an organisational strategy supported by local information and involvement (Harvey 1996). The strategy must be linked to organisational strategic plans and translated into meaningful objectives for nurses.

Senior nurses need to ensure that there is strong organisational support for improving discharge practice, and this must be explicit in order to bring about a change in culture. However, too much central control will lead to less ownership at ward level, so it is important to ensure that there is individual involvement and genuine representation. Devolution of responsibilities should be accompanied by a training strategy so that nurses are equipped to implement the changes.

The role of the senior nurse is to ensure that the training strategy is realistic and deliverable and linked to the organisational business planning process so that the need for resources is identified. Finally, the senior nurse must ensure that progress is reported, both to nurses and to the Trust Board, to maintain support and commitment.

Matrons' responsibilities

Matrons' responsibility

The 'NHS Plan' (DoH 2000) laid out the Chief Nursing Officer's (CNO's) 'Ten key roles' for nurses, of which admission and discharge was one. This was followed by a letter from Sarah Mullally (the then CNO), addressed to lead nurses in strategic health authorities and heads of nursing, clearly outlining the responsibilities of the modern matron in relation to the ten key roles.

The letter stated:

> At the Chief Nursing Officer's Annual Conference in November 2001, the Secretary of State for Health said that he expected modern matrons to report annually on progress implementing the '10 key roles'. He said this should go to their Chief Executives, who have the ability to remove organisational blocks, and also to me. (PL/CNO 2002/5)

The 2003 Department of Health publication 'Modern matrons – Improving the patient experience' lists the matron's ten key responsibilities (not to be confused with the ten key roles for nurses) as:

1. Leading by example
2. Making sure patients get quality care
3. Ensuring staffing is appropriate to patient needs
4. Empowering nurses to take on a wider range of clinical tasks
5. Improving hospital cleanliness
6. Ensuring patients' nutritional needs are met
7. Improving wards for patients
8. Making sure patients are treated with respect
9. Preventing hospital-acquired infection
10. Resolving problems for patients and their relatives by building closer relationships

Whilst discharge processes are not directly mentioned, discharge practice could be said to be part of the quality of care and clinical tasks. Ensuring that patients' nutritional needs are met, and resolving problems for patients and their relatives by building closer relationships, would arguably also reduce length of stay and expedite discharge.

There is a clear expectation that matrons will provide strong leadership and act as a link between Board-level nurses and clinical practice. Nurses at Board level have a responsibility to ensure that nursing meets Trust objectives. The role of the matron is to implement these objectives in practice. This can sometimes lead to an apparent contradiction, as the matron endeavours to improve the quality of patient care and the patient experience at the same time as supporting timely discharge. Discharging a patient quickly may not always feel like the right thing to do, as it may mean taking more risks, but it may in fact be in the best interests of the patient.

Evaluation of matrons' role

In 2004, an evaluation of the matron's role was carried out, on behalf of the Department of Health, by the Royal College of Nursing Institute and the University of Sheffield School of Nursing and Midwifery. This showed that the way in which Trusts have implemented the matron's role varies, with the number of matron posts in each organisation varying from 1 to 52. The models of working also vary, with some matrons' posts having a minimal clinical input.

The evaluation did demonstrate that most matrons' job descriptions included responsibility for discharge processes as part of their professional standard/clinical governance remit. Clearly, discharge is seen as an important part of the matron's role in many organisations. But, with competing priorities, blurred role boundaries and differing levels of authority, the impact of matrons on discharge efficiency will vary from one organisation to another.

The matron's role is to provide leadership and therefore to give the nursing team momentum and motivation. He/she should be involved in the development of an organisational strategy. The matron can then help translate this strategy into directorate plans and assist ward sisters in formulating the strategy in the form of team objectives. He/she needs to involve ward-based practitioners to determine where problems lie, identify local solutions, and ensure that ward-based practitioners receive regular feedback. The matron will also work with ward sisters to facilitate learning through experience.

The matron needs to reassure senior nurses that progress is being made, but this feedback should not be so onerous that it gets in the way of improving discharge practices. Reporting systems should always be simple and manageable.

Tables of responsibilities

Matron's responsibilities:	Board-level nurse's responsibilities:
• Translate strategy into local plans • Provide leadership • Help teams 'face reality' • Support the development of performance measures • Work with practice development teams to develop a training plan • Bring about action • Give feedback on progress to teams and Board-level nurses	• Develop a discharge strategy • Provide leadership • Support the development of performance measures • Integrate training plan into organisational business planning • Give feedback on progress to Trust Board

Bringing about action

Berwick (2003) describes three main steps that are required for improvement to take place:
- Face reality
- Seek new designs
- Involve everyone

Clinical practice considerations

'Facing reality' means identifying what needs changing, and asking: what is the gap between the current situation and what you want to achieve? 'Seeking new designs' involves acknowledging that ideas can come from anyone, and then enabling the new ideas to be implemented. 'Involving everyone' is important at each stage of the improvement or change in practice. It can be time-consuming, but the members of each clinical team need to identify what has to change in their own performance. This can sometimes be problematic, as individuals and teams will often attempt to blame others for the problem (e.g. 'Pharmacy is responsible for the delays in discharge because we have to wait so long for the tablets to be dispensed' or 'Ambulance is responsible because they don't pick up the patient on time'). Valid, believable data is important in order to persuade individuals to 'face reality'.

Maintaining the momentum

Maintaining momentum

One of the biggest difficulties in implementing new practices is maintaining their momentum. Senior nurses (both matrons and Board-level nurses) need to know that changes in practice are being implemented, that improvements in performance are being made, and that the changes are sustainable. One way to achieve this is to measure performance and put in place a robust reporting mechanism. However, the reporting mechanism must aid learning and not be seen as a punitive process, as this can have a negative impact on morale.

As Berwick (2003, p. 449) so eloquently describes it: 'The most effective route to improvement is through changing systems, not yelling at them'. The frequency of reporting required will depend on the measure being implemented. But the need for monitoring and reporting at Trust Board level must always be taken into account.

The Secretary of State for Health (PL/CNO 2002/5) put this responsibility firmly in the hands of the matron. But Board-level nurses need to recognise that some matrons need help to put these systems in place. A structured management system used across the organisation will support the monitoring of improvement and sustainability. There are various management systems that can be used, including the European Foundation for Quality Management

(EFQM) Excellence Model, Six Sigma, Lean, and Balanced Scorecard. All have been used in businesses around the world and are being adopted in healthcare organisations in the United Kingdom.

Six Sigma

Six Sigma uses statistical tools to reveal variation and implement changes to reduce the variation. Its stages are Define, Measure, Analyse, Improve, Control (DMAIC) and it is based on the Plan Do Study Act cycle, originally cited by Deming (1989). This cycle is now recommended by the Institute of Innovation and Improvement (formerly the Modernisation Agency) as a tool for change.

Applied to discharge, the Six Sigma framework requires data to be collected that relates to the patient pathway. This would highlight the elements that could be reduced/streamlined, thus reducing length of stay.

Lean

Lean is focused on work and it is about improving the flow. (In relation to discharge, this would mean reducing delays in the patient stay.) A more detailed explanation of Six Sigma and Lean is given in the NHS Institute for Innovation and Improvement publication 'Lean Six Sigma: some basic concepts' (2005).

Balanced scorecard

The balanced scorecard is a set of measures that provide a rounded picture of the improvement made. The measures are usually based around the customer or patient, finances, internal business, and innovation and learning. These categories can be adapted to suit the needs of the organisation.

EFQM Excellence Model

EFQM was formed in 1988 by the presidents of a number of major European companies. It now has over 850 members, including some healthcare organisations. The excellence model is based on the following eight concepts:

1. Results
2. Customers
3. Leadership
4. Efficient processes
5. A learning culture

The role of the practice and professional development team

6. Responsibility to the community
7. Continuous learning
8. Developing partners

(British Quality Foundation 2000)

A central part of the model is RADAR (which stands for Results, Approach, Deployment, Assessment and Review). This is what makes improvements happen.

Measuring improvement

Measuring improvement

In this chapter the focus is on using RADAR as a tool in clinical teams. It can be used as a stand-alone tool, although the principles of EFQM are that the whole business Excellence Model should be implemented to gain the most benefit. Nevertheless, using RADAR on its own is a useful starting point.

First, decide what you need to improve in relation to what you want to achieve. A number of improvements may be needed. Prioritise these and decide what you are aiming for. Involve patients and carers to help identify what needs improving (Results). Then decide how you are going to make the improvement (Approach). Having identified what you want to change and how you are going to do it, implement the changes (Deployment). Measure what you have achieved (Assessment) and learn from your progress, or lack of progress (Review).

The review might demonstrate:

- That the results were realistic or not realistic
- That the approach was appropriate or not appropriate
- That the approach was deployed effectively or not effectively

The review should take place at practice level, with the whole team, to encourage learning. Going through this process regularly allows changes to be implemented in order to achieve the desired results.

Here's an example of RADAR being applied by an individual. Let's say you decide to improve your fitness. You would like to be able to run in next year's London marathon. Your target is to complete the course in five hours (Result).

Your plan (Approach) is:

- To go to the gym every evening after work
- To eat a healthy diet
- To cut out alcohol
- To stop smoking

You do this by joining a gym, buying a vegetable steamer, a healthy eating cookery book, and nicotine patches, and by not buying alcohol (Deployment).

You measure your progress by how many minutes you can do on the running machine at the gym, the number of cigarettes you have smoked and drinks you have had, and how much weight you have lost (Assessment).

Finally, you compare your progress with your target (i.e. running the marathon in five hours) and implement changes to your approach accordingly (Review). When applied to organisational or team objectives, this methodology provides a focus for everyone and quickly shows whether or not the improvement is being made.

The table overleaf shows how RADAR can be used in relation to the discharge process.

Whatever tool you use to promote improvement and sustainability, it should:

- Support the improvement and not be too onerous
- Be understood by those who are expected to use it
- Be integrated into daily practice
- Be linked to team/organisational objectives
- Be flexible to allow changes to be made if things are not going as planned

Other questions to be considered include:

- Can you collect the data to enable you to assess where you are now and the progress you have made?
- How will you report your findings to those involved and to other key stakeholders?
- How often will you collect the data?
- Who will take responsibility for each action?
- Who do you need to involve?
- Can changes in practice be tested locally to encourage learning in the whole team?

Skills analysis

Skills analysis

Individual practitioners who take on the devolved responsibility of discharge obviously need to have the requisite skills and competencies. When implementing a change in practice, organisations often react in one of two ways. Either they offer no training

Clinical practice considerations

The discharge process RADAR

Results	Approach	Deployment	Assessment*	Review*
The discharge lounge is used for all appropriate discharges (minimum 20% of target)	• Each ward informed of target discharge lounge usage by day • Performance data shared at senior sister and directorate meetings • Action plans implemented and practice re-evaluated if targets are not consistently being met	• Refine discharge lounge targets to reflect daily target of 20% • Introduce senior sisters to targets through one-to-one sessions • Increase staff and patient awareness of the purpose and how to access the discharge lounge	Discharge lounge used 22% of target in first month and 25% in second month	Achieving above target, continue to assess each month and consider increasing target
Actual and potential discharges are identified accurately, ensuring capacity data available throughout the day	• Actual and potential discharge information identifiable within each clinical area • Qualified nurses are skilled in making these predictions • All actual and potential discharges are actioned to ensure a positive and safe outcome	• Local standard systems are developed to ensure data is clearly available • Staff skills in discharge planning and predicting are improved in conjunction with the Trust-wide discharge Training Needs Analysis project • Retrospective data is scrutinised to ensure accuracy of predictions and remedial action taken where indicated	36% wards complying	Local standard systems implemented Training not implemented, resulting in non-compliance review of training methods to be completed by end of month and changes implemented if required Predictions inaccurate due to lack of training

Based on RADAR used by Heart of England NHS Trust
The Assessment and Review are fictitious

Maintaining strategic organisational momentum

at all or they send as many staff as possible on an apparently relevant study day. Both reactions can end up wasting staff time and resources.

A more useful approach to training would begin with a skills analysis. A skills analysis identifies the gap between the level of competence the organisation requires and the level of competence employees can offer. This process means that training is tailored to organisational needs.

The skills analysis cycle

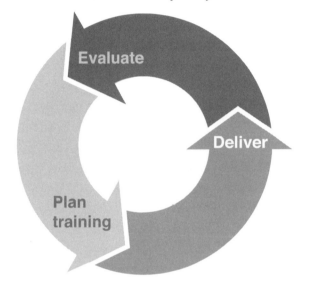

This diagram illustrates how a skills analysis should be undertaken: identify the training needs or skills gap, plan the training to meet the needs of the learner, and then decide the most appropriate methods to deliver the training. Finally, evaluation is important to ensure that the training or skills need is met.

First, it is important to decide which aspects of the discharge process each team member will be responsible for. Clarity about roles and responsibilities is key to identifying training and development needs for individuals and the team as a whole. Once you have a strategy for role development, it is possible to decide the skills and competency levels required.

'Achieving timely "simple" discharge from hospital: A toolkit for the multidisciplinary team' (DoH 2004b, pp. 41–43) includes a fact sheet on competencies for timely discharge. This includes a framework for assessing levels of competency. Skills for Health also has competencies in relation to discharge which can be found at

Clinical practice considerations

www.skillsforhealth.org.uk. Lees and Emmerson (2006) identify four aspects of discharge:

- Corporate
- Operational
- Clinical
- Nurse- or therapist-led discharges

Competencies can be identified within each of these aspects. However, the competencies should not focus solely on discharge, as some staff will also need the skills to implement and evaluate changes in practice.

Additional competencies should therefore be developed in relation to:

- Managing change
- Report writing
- Auditing
- Decision-making
- Influencing
- Knowledge of appropriate management systems

Lees and Emmerson (2006) identified 49 aspects of discharge planning for their training needs analysis tool. However, to avoid being time-consuming to complete, the tool needs to be kept as simple as possible. The skills and competence levels must be linked to organisational and team targets and should be in line with job descriptions. If job descriptions do not adequately reflect the new roles and responsibilities then they should be rewritten. (This will need to be done in consultation with Human Resources, staff representatives and the employee.)

This skills analysis process should be incorporated into the appraisal system and the personal development plan. This ensures that the training provided is linked to personal, team and organisational objectives. It also ensures that the process is linked to the 'Knowledge and Skills Framework' (DoH 2003).

The most effective way of undertaking a skills analysis is to ask individual team members to assess their own skills. Some may find this difficult and will either overestimate their ability or (more commonly) underestimate it. To help counteract this tendency, the participant can be asked to provide evidence to support their assessment. Managers should also verify the assessments and discuss any discrepancy with the individual. Individual assessments can be collated to provide information about common areas of need among the team members. This information can then be used to draw up a training plan. An example is shown below.

A sample training plan

Competency	Demonstrate excellent knowledge of the clinical condition and the investigations/interventions required	Demonstrate ability to make effective discharge decisions
Number of staff requiring training	5	10
Priority	High	High
Method of learning	Work alongside nurse specialist Follow patient through from admission to discharge	Attend session on decision-making held in-house
Method of assessment	Assessment of competence by senior nurse using assessment criteria	Self-assessment based on learning objectives
Resources	Each participant to work supernumerary status for 5 days = 25 days	10 nurses attending half-day workshop = 5 days
Responsibility	Matron	Matron
Timescales	Assessment of competence to take place within three months	Self-assessment completed within six months

A training plan should show the importance of the competence in achieving organisational objectives. It will help identify priorities for learning and therefore the most appropriate allocation of scarce resources (time and money). It will also take into account the most effective way of meeting learning needs. The planning process should be tied into the business planning/budget setting cycle so that resources can be allocated in a timely manner. The plan must also be reviewed at least annually to ensure its continuing relevance.

Clinical practice considerations

The role of the Practice and Professional Development Team

> **Practice development team responsibilities:**
> - Work with matrons and sisters to identify training needs
> - Help facilitate changes in practice
> - Provide evidence to support changes in practice
> - Help to identify current reality
> - Ensure changes are in line with the national professional agenda
> - Support the development and delivery of education
> - Provide support with the audit process
> - Form links with local educational institutions
> - Help identify sources of funding for education
> - Identify transferable skills

McCormack *et al.* (1999) describe practice development as: 'a continuous process of improvement towards increased effectiveness in patient-centred care, through the enabling of nurses and health care teams to transform the culture and context of care. It is enabled and supported by facilitators committed to a systematic, rigorous continuous process of emancipatory change'.

McCormack and Garbett (2003) identified five areas of working for Practice and Professional Development teams (P&PDTs):

1. Promoting and facilitating change
2. Research
3. Responding to external influences
4. Education
5. Audit and quality

However, nurses often see practice development as being synonymous with course attendance (Garbett 2001). Most organisations have a P&PDT, but the model and level of working will vary from one organisation to another. This will impact on the way the team works and the level of support they are able to give ward practitioners. Inevitably, this will lead to differing perceptions of the P&PDT's role.

Unsworth (2000) described practice development as:
- Facilitation through an identified source
- Planned systematic change

- Utilisation of evidence
- Responding to identified client need
- Improving services to the client
- Improving the professional's role or skills
- Improving the business or the profession or the organisation
- Improving the effectiveness of the service

He also said that it involves:

- New ways of working that lead to a direct measurable improvement in the care or service to the client
- Changes that occur as a response to a specific client need or problem
- Changes that lead to the development of effective services
- The maintenance or expansion of business/work

This can only be achieved by practice development nurses working closely with practice-based nurses. Clearly, discharge practice will not be the only area of change within an organisation, and practice development nurses may find their abilities stretched in order to meet several different needs. However, one responsibility of practice development nurses is to identify transferable skills and rationalise the way they deliver their role. Practice development nurses therefore can and should provide support to clinical teams in a number of ways.

First, the practice development nurse can help provide nurses with the evidence they need to support change. There is a perception among nurses that research is inaccessible. But this problem can be overcome with the support of clinical nurse specialists and nurse consultants (Thompson *et al.* 2001). There is no reason why practice development nurses shouldn't have some input into this role too.

As already mentioned, leadership and involvement are key to bringing about change. Pethybridge (2004) identifies the importance of multidisciplinary working in relation to discharge planning. One recommendation is to carry out 'away days' to allow teams to explore each other's roles, and to plan and identify training needs. External facilitators could be used to deliver away days. But practice development nurses may also be able to facilitate away days objectively, whilst providing an understanding of the culture and ways of working.

The practice development nurse can work with matrons and ward sisters to help identify training needs (see skills analysis,

Clinical practice considerations

pp. 85–89) and translate this into a training plan. He/she will then be able to help decide on the best ways to enable learning to take place. Traditional teaching methods may not always be the most effective, either in terms of learning or in use of resources. Releasing staff from the workplace is always a problem, and classroom teaching is not necessarily appropriate when teaching practice-based skills. A number of other methods may be preferable, including shadowing, supervision, reflection, attending ward rounds and meetings, as well as mentoring.

The P&PDT will help to present a strategic view of the input required and the cost – in terms of time and money. They will also have links with educational institutions and will be able to locate external sources of education and funding.

The audit process and its impact on practice

The audit process

The audit process is an integral part of clinical governance. Clinical governance leads in Trusts are therefore responsible for its implementation. The audit process can be used to support RADAR (see diagram below).

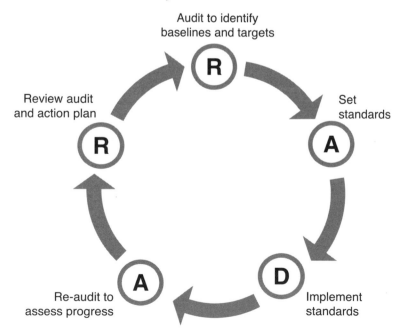

The relationship between audit and RADAR

Audit to identify
baselines and targets

Review audit
and action plan

Set
standards

Re-audit to
assess progress

Implement
standards

Maintaining strategic organisational momentum

There is evidence that auditing benefits patient care but the audit process is only successful, and only impacts on practice, if there is strong leadership. Adequate resources are also needed to carry out the audit and implement change, and expertise is required to undertake the audit (Johnston & Crombie 2000).

Trusts have clinical audit departments that may offer support to undertake an audit in relation to discharge. Most Trusts select areas of practice for audit that will impact on a high volume of patients. The areas or topics chosen are also likely to be high-risk, high-profile, and have high cost implications for the Trust. Ideally, it will be a multidisciplinary topic (Clinical Governance Support Team 2005).

Each organisation will have its own method of obtaining help from its audit department. If the audit team members are unable to offer full support for an audit, they will advise on the design of the audit form, and the gathering of data and its interpretation. Failing this, staff within the clinical team can develop the appropriate audit skills by incorporating them into their skills analysis for discharge practice (see p. 88) and subsequent training plan.

Medical staff often have an allotted time for audit but this is unlikely to be the case in any other profession. It is therefore vital that the audit is undertaken in a structured way and has a champion to lead it. The sample for the audit may be quite small to enable the audit to be carried out quickly and make the process less onerous. Nonetheless it still needs to be large enough to be representative. Clinical audit experts will be able to advise on this. As with RADAR, it may be helpful to involve patients and carers in developing the audit process and setting standards.

The Department of Health (2004) includes a fact sheet (7), which suggests areas that could be audited in relation to discharge. To establish a baseline, you may need to undertake a retrospective audit of patient records. You can then develop an audit form for staff to complete to establish current practice. Although it is recognised that patients may benefit from an audit, healthcare professionals often see the audit process as a rather unwelcome addition to their already heavy workload. Involving staff throughout the development of an audit process will make it far more likely that they will agree to undertake the work involved in carrying out the audit.

Clinical practice considerations

Conclusion

The most important factors in maintaining momentum at organisational level are strong leadership and local involvement. However, it can be hard to find a balance between centralisation and devolution, and getting it wrong may lead to a failure in implementation either at the beginning or later on (when the change in practice should have become part of everyday working).

Board-level commitment and explicit support are needed to help overcome the possible barriers to success. Matrons have been given responsibility for this, but Board-level nurses will also need to help facilitate this process. Frequent, accurate feedback about progress (or lack of progress) is vital to maintain the enthusiasm of practitioners and the support of executives. A lack of progress should not be seen negatively. Instead, it can be used to identify where further changes need to be made and to promote learning. A structured approach to identifying skills, delivering training and education, and managing and measuring the improvement made will provide a framework for successful change. Involving others, including the practice development team and the audit team, will also help to spread the workload.

References

Berwick, D.M. (2003). 'Improvement, trust, and the healthcare workforce'. *Quality and Safety in Healthcare*, **12**, 448–452.

British Quality Foundation (2000). *The Model in Practice.* London: British Quality Foundation.

Clarke, A. (2002). 'Length of in-hospital stay and its relationship to quality of care'. *Quality and Safety in Healthcare*, **11**, 209–210.

Clinical Governance Support Team (2005). *A Practical Handbook for Clinical Audit Guidance*. London: Clinical Governance Support team

Deming, W.E. (1989). *Out of the Crisis*. Cambridge, MA: MIT Press.

Department of Health (2000). 'The NHS Plan'. London: The Stationery Office.

Department of Health (2002). Professional Letter, Chief Nursing Officer, PL/CNO London: The Stationery Office.

Department of Health (2003). 'The NHS Knowledge and Skills Framework and Development Review Process'. London: The Stationery Office.

Department of Health (2004a). 'An Evaluation of the Matron's role'. The Royal College of Nursing Institute and The University of Sheffield School of Nursing and Midwifery.

Department of Health (2004b). 'Achieving timely "simple" discharge from hospital: A toolkit for the multidisciplinary team'. London: The Stationery Office.

Drake, L., Bore, J., Humm, C. & McMahon, B. (2004). 'Down with targets'. *Nursing Standard*, **19** (9), 22.

Garbett, R. & McCormack, B. (2001). 'The experience of practice development: an exploratory telephone interview study'. *Journal of Clinical Nursing*, **10** (1), 94–102.

NHS Institute for Innovation and Improvement (2005). 'Lean Six Sigma: some basic concepts'. University of Warwick.

Johnston, G., Crombie, I., Alder, E.M., Davies, H., & Millard, A. (2000). 'Reviewing audit: barriers and facilitating factors for effective clinical audit'. *Quality and Safety in Healthcare*, **9** (1), 23–36.

Lees, L. & Emmerson, K. (2006). 'Identifying discharge practice training needs'. *Nursing Standard*, **20** (29), 47–51.

McCormack, B., Manley, K., Kitson, A. & Harvey, G. (1999). 'Towards practice development – a vision in reality or a reality without vision'. *Journal of Nursing Management*, 7, 255–264.

McCormack, B. & Garbett, R. (2003). 'The characteristics, qualities and skills of practice developers'. *Journal of Clinical Nursing*, 12 (3), 317–325.

Pethybridge, J. (2004). 'How team working influences discharge planning from hospital: a study of four multidisciplinary teams in an acute hospital in England'. *Journal of Interprofessional Care*, 18, 29–40.

Steel, K., Gertman, P.M., Crescenzi, C. & Anderson, J. (2004). 'Iatrogenic illness on a general medical service at a university hospital'. *Quality and Safety in Healthcare*, 13, 76–80.

Thompson, C., McCaughan, D., Cullum, N., Sheldon, T., Mulhall, A. & Thompson, D. (2001). 'The accessibility of research-based knowledge for nurses in United Kingdom acute care settings'. *Journal of Advanced Nursing*, 36 (1), 11–22.

Unsworth, J. (2000). 'Practice development: a concept analysis'. *Journal of Nursing Management*, 8 (6), 317–326.

Chapter 6

Doctors, discharge and the interface with the multidisciplinary team

Philip Dyer and Mark Temple

Over the last 20 years, the number of NHS acute hospital beds has been reduced by 30 per cent (Pollock & Dunnigan 2000). Effective bed management is therefore a key concern for all NHS acute trusts, and length of patient stay is widely used to assess the efficiency of bed utilisation. With annual operational costs of up to a million pounds for a large acute medical ward, reducing length of stay and increasing bed occupancy rates are seen as vital tools in balancing the books. Inefficient bed utilisation, on the other hand, can have a seriously negative impact on elective services and emergency care.

For clinical staff, efficient discharge is a vital part of the hospital pathway for the individual patient. However, effective patient discharge across the whole of an acute trust is even more vital, making resources and staff available to maintain efficient service provision throughout the organisation. This makes planning discharge in advance extremely important. Patients, their carers and healthcare staff all need to be involved in discharge planning so that discharge proceeds on the planned day, delays are avoided and the use of resources (staff and bed capacity) is optimised.

Effective, timely discharge from hospital is at the core of an efficient NHS and has been the focus of a series of Department of Health publications promoting best practice. These include 'Achieving timely "simple" discharge from hospital: A toolkit for the multidisciplinary team' (DoH 2004) and 'Discharge planning: pathway, process and practice' (DoH 2003). The former discusses simple discharges and the latter is aimed at more complex discharges. More recently, the Department of Health published

Clinical practice considerations

'Emergency care briefing: modernising discharge from hospital' (Lees 2006). The aim of the paper was to provide all staff working in emergency care settings with information on the major challenges to discharge planning, key web-based links, references and simple suggestions on how to achieve best practice.

However, achieving effective, sustained changes to discharge practice requires an understanding of the many facets of the discharge process, particularly the professional responsibilities of the healthcare staff involved in both simple and complex discharges.

Simple and complex discharges

Simple and complex discharge

Hospital discharges are described as fitting into one of two categories: simple or complex. Simple discharges make up at least 80 per cent of all discharges and are the norm in patients where a self-limiting condition has responded to treatment. Consequently, it is usually the response to treatment that dictates the time when the patient will be discharged. Those patients whose discharge is classified as simple do not require major additional post-discharge support and care arrangements that are likely to influence the timing of discharge. The Department of Health discharge 'toolkit' (2004) defines simple discharges as those patients who will usually be discharged to their own homes and have simple ongoing care needs which do not require complex planning and delivery.

Up to 20 per cent of all discharges are complex discharges. However, in certain specialised hospital settings (such as an acute care of the elderly ward) the majority of discharges may be complex. Complex discharge patients are more likely to:

- Be discharged to a setting other than their own home (e.g. a nursing home or residential home)
- Have complex ongoing health and social care needs, requiring detailed assessment, planning and delivery by the multidisciplinary team
- Have their date of discharge determined by the speed at which arrangements to meet ongoing care needs can be set up outside hospital

For every patient, the objective is to be discharged from acute hospital care as soon as the patient no longer requires that level of care. 'Timely discharge' thus means that the patient is discharged home or to an ongoing level of care (such as a nursing home) as soon as they are clinically stable and fit for discharge.

Discharge decision-making – the doctor and the multidisciplinary team

The doctor and the team

Discharge from hospital should be planned and implemented by the multidisciplinary team (MDT). The team will include medical and nursing staff, allied health professionals (AHPs) and social workers. The more complex the discharge, the larger the number of team members that are likely to be involved, and the more planning and communication will be required between the team members, the patient, carers and other agencies or staff. The effectiveness of the MDT's working practices will be demonstrated by the timeliness of the discharge, the quality of the arrangements for care post-discharge, and the level of understanding of the patient and their carers throughout the discharge process.

The MDT needs a clinical leader and this role is commonly filled by the consultant in charge of the patient's care. The consultant in charge is the member of the team with the clearest medico-legal responsibility for all aspects of the patient's care while in hospital. This responsibility is a major reason why the consultant conventionally assumes the role of team leader. However, the consultant may not be the team member with the best skills to coordinate arrangements for a complex discharge. Consultants who recognise this delegate the lead discharge role to another team member. In designated nurse- or therapist-led wards the discharge process is led exclusively by non-medical staff.

Doctors have three crucial areas of involvement in the discharge process. These are:

- Conducting ward rounds
- Recording (medical) management plans in the case notes
- Participating in the multidisciplinary team (MDT) meetings

Ward rounds and clinical decision-making

Ward rounds

Ward rounds play a pivotal part in delivering high-quality hospital-based care. Ward rounds should be multi-professional, enabling doctors and other healthcare professionals to develop an

Clinical practice considerations

integrated plan of care. According to Manias & Street (2000), the goals of the ward round in both medical and surgical practice include:

- Enhancing the quality of care
- Improving communication
- Addressing patient concerns and problems
- Planning and evaluating treatment

Multi-professional training and education are also enhanced by the ward round.

Little is known, however, about the origins of the ward round and variations in ward round practice. The ward round often provides the only opportunity for genuine multi-professional working. The benefits of multi-professional clinical practice are not confined to acute ward settings but are also enshrined in good practice initiatives such as the care programme approach or CPA (Easton & Oyebode 1996).

In medical practice, attempts have been made to define ward round standards (Plume 1985) but these guidelines are likely to be outdated. Medical and nursing trainees receive virtually no training in relation to the objectives of the ward round, how to participate in it, how it should be structured and how to get the desired outcomes. Lees *et al.* (2006) listed the key components of a good post-take ward round and these can be applied to all types of ward rounds. These generic components include:

1. Information gathering
2. Engaging the medical team and MDT in the ward round discussions and decisions that arise
3. Assimilation of information
4. Teaching/educating all members of the MDT and patients
5. Making decisions based on the information available
6. Listening to and involving the patients in the decisions about their care
7. Giving verbal explanation of the decision to all members of the ward round, including patients
8. Providing a written record of the decision (i.e. a management/discharge plan, preferably using some sort of pre-written proforma)
9. Empowering nursing staff and other members of the MDT to implement agreed actions and problem-solve after the ward round is finished
10. Reviewing progress of previous ward round decisions

Doctors, discharge and the interface

All participating staff should be aware of the start time and likely duration of the ward round in advance. The agreed timing and duration of the round should take into account the likely nature and number of patients to be reviewed and the availability of the MDT.

Although medical and nursing staff are the core participants, for a variety of reasons ward rounds may often be conducted solely by medical staff. If doctors start rounds at erratic times, without prior warning, there is little opportunity for other staff to attend. Limited nursing staff numbers on busy acute wards also prevent nurses from participating in several ward rounds when these are conducted simultaneously on the same ward by different medical teams. The lack of multidisciplinary input in ward rounds has been noted in psychiatry (Rix & Sheppard 2003) but it is also common in both medicine and surgery.

In the context of a busy acute medical and surgical ward, routine participation in ward rounds by nurses requires leadership, a culture of prioritising multi-professional working and considerable consistent effort. It is all too easy for ward rounds staffed solely by doctors to become the norm. If this happens, nurses will lose a key opportunity to participate in clinical decision-making affecting their patients.

The effectiveness of decision-making on 'doctors only' rounds depends on the information available from the case notes or from the patient and the quality of communication with other healthcare staff. Poor communication is a frequent problem. For instance, there may be a hurried handover of major decisions made to a ward nurse by the most junior member of the medical team at the end of a doctor's ward round. Doctors frequently fail to discuss discharge plans on rounds, and the entry in the clinical notes relating to the round may bear little relation to the issues discussed (Lees & Holmes 2005).

'Doctors only' rounds disenfranchise other members of the MDT, who cannot then share information with medical staff, or raise issues of concern or points requiring clarification, or participate in treatment and discharge decisions. Patients report that they don't understand what is said by doctors on ward rounds and they rely on other members of the team to explain management and discharge decisions made on ward rounds (Lees and Holmes 2005).

Clinical practice considerations

During a multi-professional ward round, every member of the MDT should be aware of their role. The skill, experience and manner of the senior clinician, often a consultant, when conducting the round is critical in maintaining focus and optimal input from all participants.

Pathak *et al.* (2000) observed the individual skills of 12 senior consultants with more than 10 years' experience in neurosurgical practice at three different university hospitals during their ward rounds. The ward rounds were reported to show evidence of good productivity and flexibility among 92 per cent and 75 per cent of the consultants respectively. Pleasantness of the climate was reported to be above average on rounds conducted by just 50 per cent of the consultants, with poor objectivity shown by 42 per cent of consultants.

In addition, 42 per cent of the consultants were not consistently well understood. Only half the consultants were reported to use words and phrases fitting the circumstances of the round. A total of 42 per cent spoke unnecessarily between discussions and introduced the problems of the patient poorly to the MDT, and only 33 per cent managed to use humour effectively. Pathak *et al.* concluded that conducting ward rounds in neurosurgical practice needs a holistic approach, with motivation, planning, leadership skills and a structured curriculum to fulfil objectives. The range of these failings emphasises the variety of skills required by the consultant conducting the round. And it is likely that many of these failings are common to ward rounds wherever they occur.

High-quality communication skills are therefore crucial to the effectiveness of the ward round. Ultimately, the consultant needs to develop – with the rest of the MDT – a plan for the management and discharge of the patient that is comprehensive but also easy to follow.

One area of concern has been the tendency for the consultant in charge to dominate the MDT on ward rounds, resulting in an 'impotent' team. Gair (2001) observed team practice in a care of the elderly setting and reported a lower than expected level of medical dominance. Gair related this finding to the consultant's own views on the nature of rehabilitation, leading to a consensus among team members as to the purpose of geriatric assessment, and to a high level of team stability. He concluded that reducing the level of medical dominance encourages all team members to contribute, and thus enhances patient care.

Doctors, discharge and the interface

More training for doctors in team skills was considered beneficial, including inter-professional training. Gair stressed the importance of the consultant avoiding monopolisation of the conversation and recommended inviting comments through questions. Encouraging participation by asking open questions, such as 'What does everyone think about what has been said?' or 'Can anyone add something more or some other points that need to be mentioned?', will lead to a more inclusive ward round and at the same time test the strength of a point or view.

Teaching is an integral part of the consultant's role, and the consultant should help to create a learning climate during ward rounds for the MDT. In 'The doctor as teacher' the General Medical Council states that 'all doctors have a professional obligation to contribute to the education and training of others' and that 'every doctor should be prepared to oversee the work of less experienced colleagues' (GMC 1999).

Interdisciplinary teaching rounds have been shown to promote more efficient patient care by providing an opportunity for enhanced communication among healthcare professionals (Felten 1997). The consultant ward round is a setting where experiential learning occurs and this is highly valued by trainees. Talbot (2000) found the ward round to be a very useful teaching resource according to questionnaire responses given by 500 Senior House Officers (SHOs) in North Trent. The trainees found the ward rounds particularly useful when learning professional attributes and skills but less useful for learning clinical science principles and management strategies. In relation to discharge planning, the ward round provides an important opportunity for senior staff to embed good discharge practice as a core responsibility of junior medical and nursing staff.

There is great potential for shared learning within the hospital environment, and this may provide an extension to experiential and self-directed learning (Gibson 2000). Reeves *et al.* (2000) undertook a pilot project for pre-registration house officers and newly qualified nurses, focusing on areas of the hospital service that could be improved (including discharge planning and intravenous drug administration). The participants were asked to work together to solve problems based on clinical scenarios. The study concluded that such sessions encouraged collaboration between members of the clinical team to the benefit of patient

Clinical practice considerations

care and addressed some important clinical governance issues.

Some authors have expressed concern about shared learning, stating that healthcare professions are distinct from each other and should remain separate (Farmer 1995, Castledine 1999). On balance, the current literature supports exploring uni-professional and multi-professional shared learning, the perceived benefits being improved interdisciplinary working, improved communication, and acquisition of new skills and knowledge.

A study by Davis and Dent (1994) showed that medical students learn from attending both outpatient clinics and ward rounds. The learning experience was reported to be better in the outpatient clinic. However, the students did not make full use of the learning potential of either. Consultant psychiatrists surveyed about their ward rounds reported that these were largely a compromise between professional efficiency and patient satisfaction, with little mention made of any educational element (Hodgson 2005).

Although ward rounds are recognised learning opportunities for medical students and junior doctors there has, until recently, been little emphasis on acquiring the skills to conduct a successful ward round. However, the reform of postgraduate medical education embodied in the Modernising Medical Careers initiative (Operational Framework for Foundation Training, DoH 2005) has helped focus attention on neglected areas of junior doctor training.

An initiative in Worthing relating to best practice on the post-take ward round has been highlighted on the modernising medical careers website (www.mmc.nhs.uk/pages/resources/info-for-trainers#Post). Here, Dr Gordon Caldwell has incorporated a standardised instant assessment and feedback process into the routine post-take ward round. This has greatly improved the effectiveness of the post-take ward round and also offers learning points and objectives for both trainee and trainer. The time invested in assessment of the ward round has yielded rewards, including quicker ward rounds. The time saved can then be used for more teaching or for increased communication with patients.

It is thus essential that protected time for a reflective element is included in the timetables of both teachers and learners if this mode of learning is to be effective. At present, the lack of allocated time for reflection is a major barrier to maximising opportunities for experiential learning in the clinical environment of the NHS.

Doctors, discharge and the interface

Nurse participation in ward rounds

Despite the tools, protocols and guidance, described earlier in this chapter, that are available to empower nurses to discharge patients, nurse-led discharge is still relatively rare. Where multidisciplinary ward rounds occur routinely, the criteria for discharge need to be clearly stated, together with the responsibility of members of the MDT to ensure that these criteria are met and the discharge implemented. Pockets of good practice have sprung up in many parts of the NHS; however, these are the exceptions rather than the norm. For good discharge practice to flourish consistently, decision-making skills (critical to the ward round process) and accountability need to be continually reinforced in the practice setting, implementing the theory taught at universities.

Decision-making is fundamental to discharge planning, yet there appears to be some reluctance among nursing staff to take on this role. This may be because of competing clinical priorities, a feeling that decisions about discharge should be left to medical staff, or simply a reluctance to make key decisions about discharge. The decision-making process requires confidence, and confidence can only be gained through knowledge and experience. The structure supporting nurses and their individual accountability is provided by the 2004 'Nursing and Midwifery code of professional conduct: standards for conduct, performance and ethics' (www.nmc-uk.org), which states that 'You are personally accountable for your practice and any decisions to act or not act' (NMC 2004). This means that nurses are answerable for their actions and omissions, regardless of advice or directions from another professional.

Ward rounds that occur without regular nursing representation risk being viewed by nurses solely as a doctors' task and a source of inconvenience. In these circumstances, on the few occasions that nurses do participate they may feel undervalued and are likely to adopt a passive or reactive role. Both nursing staff and medical staff need to view the ward round as a vital aid to decision-making during the patient pathway. The ward round should therefore be truly multidisciplinary, with all members of the MDT actively involved in discharge planning and implementation. Persistent failure by nurses to participate in ward rounds undermines nurses' clinical role, erodes their skills, impedes effective MDT communication, and ultimately reduces the quality of patient care.

Clinical practice considerations

Recording management and discharge plans during the ward round

The ward round is the main clinical decision-making period for patients in the ward. Decisions made need to be recorded in the patient's clinical record clearly and accurately. However, the pressure to move on to review the next patient leaves little time available to record management plans for each patient in their case notes. Recording decisions in the case notes is often delegated to the most junior doctor on the round. These junior doctors may have limited understanding of the importance of the decisions made. They may also have the least experience of recording salient points rapidly in the case notes.

In discharge planning terms the effectiveness of the ward round depends on all members of the MDT having a clear understanding of the agreed discharge plan and their role in relation to it. The entry in the case notes informs all the MDT members (not just those attending the ward round) about the plan and their role in delivering it. However, several steps are required to get the case note entry right (Lees & Holmes 2005). First, the discharge plan needs to be discussed on the round, then discharge decisions have to be made, and finally these decisions need to be summarised accurately and legibly in the case notes.

This may sound simple but maintaining high standards of clinical documentation remains a problem, despite the emphasis put on its importance by professional bodies and medical legal defence organisations. Fernando and Siriwardena (2001) found that junior doctors on a surgical ward round frequently failed to document the consultants' clinical findings and management decisions. In addition, information given to patients by consultants regarding clinical findings and planned treatment was recorded in a median of only 6 per cent of consultations.

The use of a standardised proforma on ward rounds has been shown to improve documentation. Thompson *et al.* (2004) looked at the documentation during ward rounds before and after the introduction of a proforma. The proforma led to a significant improvement in the documentation of diagnosis, management plan, prophylaxis for deep vein thrombosis, and resuscitation status, all of which were felt to have a considerable impact on patient care. Doctors found this proforma straightforward, user-friendly, and useful for clinical practice. Compliance was enhanced by its inclusion in the patient admission pack. Other health professionals, especially nurses, found it a useful reference document when they received a new patient on the ward.

Providing an estimated date of discharge

Estimating discharge date

Providing a clear estimated date of discharge (EDD) can be seen as a critical element in the multidisciplinary discharge planning process. The objectives of discharge planning include providing the patient and carers with advance information on the timing of discharge and arrangements for post-discharge care and follow-up. Good discharge planning also requires development of an effective post-discharge care strategy with healthcare staff. In addition, it should ensure the optimal use of expensive resources (particularly hospital bed capacity and staff time).

The Department of Health discharge 'toolkit' (DoH 2004) recommends that the date of expected discharge should be estimated at the earliest opportunity after the patient's admission. However, to assess the EDD accurately, the diagnosis needs to be reasonably secure. Key assessments by the MDT also have to be available and there needs to have been sufficient time to observe the patient's level of stability and response to treatment. In practice, the post-take ward round conducted by a consultant together with the rest of the MDT, within 12 to 24 hours of the patient's admission, therefore often provides the first practical opportunity to determine the EDD (Lees *et al.* 2006).

Although the post-take ward round is the natural time for decisions to be made about the likely length of hospital stay, doctors seem reluctant to commit to an EDD. In our experience, the clinical entries by medical staff on the post-take ward round focus on clinical findings, results of tests and likely diagnosis, and planned further investigations. The estimated length of stay in hospital is frequently not considered by medical staff, despite this being a leading concern of patients and the major cost in relation to in-patient services. Based on a survey of in-patients, Lees andHolmes (2005) highlighted patients' concerns about discharge and the fact that doctors are poor at providing this information.

It is not clear why doctors are often so reluctant to provide information on EDD. It may be linked to the unstructured nature of

Clinical practice considerations

many consultant-led ward rounds, the lack of training on making rounds effective, absence of multidisciplinary representation, or excessive emphasis by senior medical staff on the challenges of diagnosis and treatment rather than predicted time in hospital.

Some patients admitted as emergencies may have complex discharge requirements. For instance, they may need multiple assessments by therapists and social workers, and this will make it difficult to give an EDD. However, the reluctance to give an EDD also occurs when doctors are well placed to provide it – for example, for patients on a medical pathway in which the duration of hospital stay relates to the timing of medical investigations and the response to treatment.

Lees *et al.* (2006) introduced a simple discharge planning summary label for completion by doctors on the post-take ward round. A key element of this label was to prompt a routine EDD for all patients admitted to an emergency admission ward. An EDD had to be completed for all patients, with a simple tick box response for those predicted as 'same day' or 'within 24 hours'. For patients with an EDD longer than 24 hours, the label prompted responses about key in-patient referrals or investigations required and the predicted admission pathway, e.g. transfer to general medical or specialist medical ward.

An audit of the first 50 labels used revealed that only 6 had an EDD entered. One of the initial reasons for the labels was to prompt and summarise decision-making when a nurse was unable to attend the post-take ward round. However, it was recognised that this acted at best as a memory jogger, and the requirement for a nurse to join the ward round remains crucial. On the basis of the initial audit the label evolved into a colour-coded A4 sheet, with space for text routinely recorded by medical staff on clinical findings and investigation results in addition to EDD information. This post-take ward round record sheet is now used all the time on the admission ward, with the intention that completing all the prompted sections will become accepted practice.

The discharge planning label audit carried out on our admission ward (Lees *et al.* 2006) highlighted extremely poor completion of the EDD by junior doctors even when this was prompted by a simple tick box response. It is important to understand the reasons for this. Although the audit did not address this, our suggestions include:

- In the absence of any clear recommended practice medical staff tend to 'do their own thing'.
- Doctors do not like to conform.
- Some doctors may feel that providing an EDD exposes them to criticism if the estimate then turns out to be incorrect.
- Some doctors feel that providing an EDD will require them to spend more time discussing the management plan with patients and relatives, including time taken 'fine tuning' the EDD on successive rounds (Lees & Holmes, 2005).
- Doctors dislike the uncertainty of stating an EDD.
- Some doctors take the view that 'Discharge of a patient will occur when I have finished with their care.'
- Doctors fail to recognise the importance of EDD in relation to the quality of patient care, length of stay and bed capacity.

For the EDD process to work, doctors must feel that the decision on the discharge date is important in the management of their patients. The decision must also be seen to generate an appropriate response (i.e. all staff need to work towards the stated EDD for the benefit of the patient).

Implementing discharge

Implementing discharge

Planning discharge is a fundamental component of all ward rounds. Nevertheless, once a discharge is agreed, the process should proceed, irrespective of the timing of the next routine ward round. All members of the MDT not only need to be aware of their role in discharge but should also be empowered to implement discharge. The ability to discharge patients out of hours and during weekends must be maintained, independently of medical staff input. Nursing staff, in particular, need to be confident about taking the lead role in ensuring that the patient leaves hospital promptly and safely.

One of the Chief Nursing Officer's 'ten key roles' for nurses in 'The NHS Plan' (DoH 2000) is admitting and discharging patients with specified conditions, supported by agreed protocols. To achieve this, however, protocols must be written that incorporate clear discharge criteria. Doctors are familiar with writing and following protocols for the management of certain conditions. But they appear to be less comfortable with specifying the criteria that would allow patients to be discharged, particularly when this occurs without medical review on the day of discharge.

In emergency care there is great emphasis on the criteria determining whether or not the patient requires hospital admission, but little on the criteria indicating the point at which the patient can safely return to the community. This may in part relate to an understandable emphasis on the patient presenting as an emergency, rather than when in a recuperating phase. However, other reasons may include: difficulties in predicting response to treatment (particularly in elderly patients with multiple co-morbidity); junior doctors' reluctance to discharge patients from the safe environment of an acute ward; and consultants' reluctance to relinquish a powerful mechanism to control the individual patient's pathway and related resources.

In elective surgical practice, protocols routinely include criteria for discharge – probably partly because of the much more predictable in-patient course in these selected patient groups. However, for patients presenting as emergencies, effective guidelines are available. For instance, the British Thoracic Society has produced comprehensive, evidenced-based but nevertheless straightforward discharge criteria for community-acquired pneumonia that can be easily applied by nursing staff (BTS 2004). The unwillingness to write or adopt these pre-specified criteria therefore appears to be the limiting factor, rather than the criteria themselves. This is a problem that needs to be addressed.

Discharge – the future

Discharge – the future

The process of discharging patients is a vitally important but frequently neglected aspect of healthcare. In this chapter we have shown that medical decision-making may be arbitrary; discharge practice is often not taught, reviewed or standardised; and the involvement of the multidisciplinary team is frequently inconsistent. Elwyn *et al.* (2005) summed up the risks of adverse events and errors during discharge with the warning: 'Avoid hospitals if you can, but if you can't take additional care when leaving'.

In the United States, InterQual (www.interqual.com/IQSite), a comprehensive software package, has been developed by McKesson to support the clinical review and discharge of patients. The software determines the appropriate level of care required for each patient according to the severity of their illness and the intensity of service they are receiving. InterQual also generates criteria that can be used to prompt discharge planning. For example, it may flag a patient likely to be suitable for discharge the next day, on the basis of clinical criteria relating to reducing severity of illness, following treatment for pneumonia.

InterQual clinical decision support tools are developed or reviewed annually in the light of evidence-based research literature. They are also validated by a large pool of clinicians before being circulated to more than 3,000 healthcare facilities in the USA.

A prominent feature of in-patient management in the USA is a much more assertive approach to discharge planning. This is linked to a much wider range of alternatives to acute in-patient care than in the NHS. As a result, length of stay (LOS) in acute hospitals in the USA is markedly shorter than in the NHS, with major implications for healthcare costs. This has recently been demonstrated in a comparison with Kaiser Permanente (KP), an integrated healthcare organisation based in California, delivering a comparable range of services to 8 million members. KP, founded in 1945, is roughly the same age as the NHS and represents a model of healthcare in the USA similar to the NHS.

In a landmark paper in 2002, Feachem *et al.* compared the costs and performance of the NHS with those of KP's California region. The per capita costs of the two systems, adjusted for differences in benefits and population characteristics, were similar to within 10 per cent. However age-adjusted rates of use of acute hospital services in KP were less than one-third of those in the NHS. There were nearly four times the number of acute bed days per 1,000 population in the NHS than in Kaiser. This reflected major differences in the management of admissions, length of stay and discharge practice.

KP bases their management of bed resources on an organisation-wide care facilitation strategy, supported by InterQual. InterQual drives the process of discharge planning through care facilitators, who track each patient's hospital journey and ensure that they are discharged when their assessment indicates that they do not require an acute hospital bed. The care facilitators are nurses with at least two years' clinical experience who manage a caseload of about 25 patients each.

Clinical practice considerations

InterQual is also used in KP to assess the appropriateness of every emergency hospital admission, and to encourage the Emergency Department to search for alternatives to admission. There is considerable interest in the use of software linked to care facilitation in the UK. Northumbria Healthcare Acute Trust have been using the InterQual criteria and care facilitation for over four years, and this Trust has evidence of reduced lengths of stay which compare very favourably with NHS averages. Our own Heart of England Acute Foundation Trust has recently commenced a pilot project using InterQual.

The use of validated evidence-based software, such as InterQual, to track acute hospital in-patients, linked with care facilitators/discharge coordinators, offers an immensely powerful tool to standardise and prompt discharge planning. This type of system can also reduce the use of resources and lessen the risks of abrupt change to the patient's level of care inherent in discharge from an acute hospital bed.

However, perhaps the most important point about clinical decision-making tools such as InterQual is that their use can provide extensive objective information on numbers of patients inappropriately admitted to, or remaining in, acute hospital care because it can be shown that their severity of illness does not require care in an acute hospital setting. All too often within the NHS acute hospital beds provide the setting for care that could be provided elsewhere.

A new emphasis on creating alternatives to acute hospital care is required in the NHS to optimise patient care and free up acute hospital beds for patients who really need them. The focus must be on admitting patients to acute hospital care only when this is required. For those patients who are admitted, safe and carefully coordinated discharge to a suitable care setting must occur just as soon as the patient no longer requires acute hospital care. The widespread use of an evidence-based, clinical decision-making tool in the NHS, such as InterQual, would play a large part in this. It would drive joint planning and investment with primary care, which would catalyse and sustain tailored care pathways that are patient-centred and evidence-based.

References

British Thoracic Society (2004 update). 'BTS guidelines for the management of community acquired pneumonia in adults'. (www.brit-thoracic.org/guidelines)

Caldwell, G. 'Post-take ward round assessment and feedback process' (www.mmc.nhs.uk/pages/resources/info-for-trainers)

Castledine, G. (1999). 'A nursing "peace" v. medical "war" model'. *British Journal of Nursing*, 8, 62.

Davis, M.H. & Dent, J.A. (May 1994). 'Comparison of student learning in the out-patient clinic and ward round'. *Medical Education*, 28 (3), 208–212.

Department of Health (2000). 'The NHS Plan'. London: The Stationery Office.

The Department of Health (2003). 'Discharge from hospital: Pathway, process and practice'. London: The Stationery Office.

Department of Health (2004). 'Achieving timely "simple" discharge from hospital: A toolkit for the multidisciplinary team'. London: The Stationery Office.

Department of Health (2005). 'Operational framework for foundation training: Modernising Medical Careers'. London: The Stationery Office.

Easton, C. & Oyebode, F. (1996). 'Care management. Administrative demands of care programme approach'. *British Medical Journal*, 312,1540.

Elwyn, G., Foster, A. & Freeman, G. (27 July 2005). 'Mind the gap: the risk of adverse events and errors during patient discharge'. (www.saferhealthcare.org.uk/IHI/Topics/DischargingPatients/WhatWeKnow/)

Farmer, E. (1995). 'Medicine and nursing: a marriage for the 21st century'. *British Journal of Nursing*, 4, 793–794.

Feachem, R.G.A., Sekhri, N.K. & White, K.L. (2002). 'Getting more for their dollar: a comparison of the NHS with California's Kaiser Permanente'. *British Medical Journal*, 234, 135–141.

Felten, S., Cady, N., Metzler, M. *et al.* (1997). 'Implementation of collaborative practice through interdisciplinary rounds on a general surgery service'. *Nursing Case Management*, 2 (3), 122–126.

Fernando, K.J. & Siriwardena, A.K. (2001). 'Standards of documentation of the surgeon-patient consultation in current surgical practice'. *British Journal of Surgery*, 88, 309–312.

Gair, G. (2001). 'Medical dominance in multidisciplinary teamwork: a case study of discharge decision-making in a geriatric assessment unit'. *Journal of Nursing Management*, 9 (1), 3–11.

Clinical practice considerations

General Medical Council (1999). 'The doctor as teacher'. GMC.

Gibson, D.R. & Campbell, R.M. (2000). 'The role of cooperative learning in the training of junior hospital doctors: a study of paediatric senior house officers.' *Medical Teacher*, 22, 297–300.

Hodgson, R., Jamal, A. & Gayathri, B. (2005). 'A survey of ward round practice'. *Psychiatric Bulletin*, 29, 171–173.

Lees, L. (2006) 'Emergency Care Briefing Paper: Modernising discharge from Hospital'. National Electronic Library for Health. (http://libraries.nelh.nhs.uk/emergency/viewResource.asp?uri = http per cent3A//libraries.nelh.nhs.uk/common/resources/ per cent3Fid per cent3D63696&categoryID = 1414)

Lees, L., Allen, G. & O'Brien, D. (2006). 'Using post-take ward rounds to facilitate simple discharge'. *Nursing Times*, 102 (18), 28–30.

Lees, L. & Holmes, C. (2005), 'Estimating date of discharge at ward level: a pilot study'. *Nursing Standard*, 17, 40–43.

Manias, E. & Street, A. (2000). 'Nurse doctor interactions during critical care ward rounds'. *Journal of Clinical Nursing*, 10, 442–450.

Nursing and Midwifery Council (2004). 'The NMC code of professional conduct: standards for conduct, performance and ethics'. London: NMC. (www.nmc-uk.org/)

Pathak, A., Pathak, N. & Kak, V. (2000) 'Ideal ward round making in neurosurgical practice'. *Neurology India*, 48, 216–222.

Pollock, A. & Dunnigan, M. (2000). 'Beds in the NHS'. *British Medical Journal*, 320, 461–462.

Reeves, S., Freeth, R. & Wood, D. (2000) 'A joint learning venture between new nurses and junior doctors'. *Nursing Times*, 96 (38), 39–40.

Rix, S. & Sheppard, G. (2003). 'Acute wards: problems and solutions: Implementing real change in acute inpatient care– more than just bringing in the builders'. *Psychiatric Bulletin*, 27, 108–111.

Talbot, M. (2000). 'Professional modeling: a questionnaire study of junior doctors' attitudes to aspects of experiential learning on the hospital ward round'. *Medical Education*, 34, 312–315.

Thompson, A.G., Jacob, K., Fulton, J. *et al.* (2004). 'Do post-take ward round proformas improve communication and influence quality of patient care?' *Postgraduate Medical Journal*, 80, 675–676.

Chapter 7

The nurse's role in facilitating complex discharge

Siân Wade

This chapter focuses on issues related to the effective discharge of individuals with complex care needs. Discharge planning is a routine feature of healthcare systems. The aim is to reduce hospital lengths of stay and unplanned re-admission, and improve the coordination of services following discharge. This should help to bridge the gap between hospital and place of discharge (Shepperd *et al.* 2004), and ensure a smooth transfer to the patient's home or a new setting.

Ideally, this planning should form an integral part of the holistic care plan, including an estimated date of discharge and plans for the necessary services required for ongoing care. For a successful outcome, a team and whole systems approach is absolutely essential. However, the role of nurses is often central, and their role will therefore receive particular emphasis.

The key principles of complex discharge are:
- Effective and timely discharge of individuals with complex care needs is important if their quality of life is to be promoted and if effective use of resources is to be maximised.
- Discharge planning for those with complex care needs usually occurs within a global context, involving multiple ongoing and underlying healthcare and social care needs. Care arrangements, which form a key component in the continuity of community care, must therefore be put in place before successful transfer or discharge to another service or home can occur.
- Effective discharge of those with complex discharge requirements requires a whole systems approach.

Clinical practice considerations

- Effective discharge places the individual at the centre of the discharge process, promoting continuity of care through adequate information and communication flow between patients, carers and services so as to ensure optimum outcomes for individuals.
- The effective discharge of those with complex care needs is both a challenging and skilled process, requiring staff to have grasped the key principles and to have developed sophisticated skills.

Social factors

Social factors

Today's increased life expectancy and improved healthcare mean that people with lifelong or ongoing health problems have a much greater chance of surviving and living longer. As such, they are more likely to have complex care needs. It is estimated that 17.5 million people in the UK have some form of long-term condition, i.e. about 6 out of 10 adults (DoH 2005a), or 30 per cent of the population. Nearly half of these people have more than one condition, and the percentage of those over 65 years old with a long-term condition is expected to double by 2030 (DoH 2005a).

The World Health Organisation (WHO) has estimated that long-term conditions will be the leading cause of disability by 2020. Further analysis shows that 80 per cent of time, energy and resources of healthcare staff and care services tend to be invested in 20 to 30 per cent of the population – those with complex care needs (CSIP 2004/5, DoH 2005a). Hence there has been a growing emphasis on finding ways to meet the needs of this client group (DoH 2005a, 2005b, 2006).

The social context in which people are ageing or developing complex care needs today has changed a great deal. Lasslett (1989) and Stearns (1976) both assert that families are no less caring today than in the past. However, the patterns of modern family life present a real challenge in terms of providing support and care. There are smaller and much more complex extended family and social networks, described by Bengston *et al.* (1990) as 'beanpole families'. Increasingly, siblings and partners involved in helping to provide care are themselves ageing or disabled. In addition, people frequently move to different parts of the country in search of work. This has led to disparate, far-flung networks that strain the ability of those involved to provide extensive care. Changing patterns in marriage, divorce and relationships can also weaken family ties and reduce commitment to care for elderly or disabled relatives. All these factors combine to present a major challenge for nurses, as well as other health and social care professionals, who are planning complex discharge.

Recognising the moral imperative

The moral imperative

It has never been so vital to ensure that the needs of individuals with complex care requirements are effectively and efficiently met within health and social care settings or services (DoH 2005a). From a political perspective, it is crucial to meet these needs, especially in view of the reduction in beds, the issues involving effective capacity management and use of resources (DoH 2005a), and the enormous debts incurred by the NHS in recent years. Similarly, from the carer's perspective, it is crucially important to ensure that patients are cared for by the right staff, with the right skills, at the right time. Even more vital, however, from a quality of life perspective, is the moral and ethical imperative of ensuring that the care of those with complex care needs is maximised within the constraints and resources available and takes place, wherever possible, in the community (Annells 2004, Hainsworth 2005, Sargent 2006, DoH 2005a, DoH 2006).

Traditionally, discharge has been associated with 'going home from hospital'. However, with changes in healthcare and social care, and the increasingly acute care available in district general hospitals, acute wards often focus less on discharge and more on assessment, treatment and intervention for those with complex needs. These individuals are often transferred on to a less acute setting or service, such as a specialist or rehabilitation ward, intermediate care, or transitional care for their ongoing care needs to be met. It is therefore not unusual for discharge planning to be deferred until the patient reaches this service. Hence in an acute setting the nurse's skills may be centred around transfer of care, rather than planning the patient's complex discharge.

Clinical practice considerations

Strategies to enhance effective discharge

Effective discharge

Measures to resolve bed capacity problems and length of stay issues have seen the introduction of a whole systems approach in many localities. This approach utilises many strategies to expedite the appropriate flow and discharge of patients, including those strategies listed in the table below.

Strategies used in a whole systems discharge approach
• Use of clinical care pathways
• Theory of constraints
• Effective knowledge and care (coordination)
• Chronic disease management programmes
• Availability of post-acute services
• Access to community support services for both health and personal care needs

Care pathways

Care pathways have a very valuable part to play in relation to the patient's journey through hospital, but they do tend to be disease-focused (Ellis & Johnson 1997, Middleton & Roberts 2000). The potential of care pathways in helping those patients with more complex needs, particularly where multiple pathology is present, is perhaps less clear. And nurses working in the field of complex discharge planning tend to have little exposure to using care pathways, perhaps partly because of their specificity. However, as Wade (2004) argues, much can be learnt from the principles of care pathways that is relevant to this group of patients. Care pathways help to ensure that care is organised, timely and focused, using evidence-based practice, providing the clinical record, and enhancing the identification of variances and risks (Oliver 2006). The requirement for multidisciplinary collaboration also aids timely involvement and continuous review of care.

Social and chronic healthcare needs

Healthcare needs

Discharge planning for those with complex care needs usually occurs within a wider context, involving multiple ongoing and underlying healthcare and social care needs. Care arrangements must therefore be put in place before successful transfer or discharge to another service or home can occur (Bull & Kane 1996). If these arrangements have not been made by the time the patient is ready to be discharged the consequences may be lasting and sometimes even fatal (Annells 2004). In such cases of delayed discharge, the health of the patient is often severely challenged, with compromised functional reserve, increased risk of iatrogenesis (Illich 1975), hospital-acquired infection (Gould 2002) and/or age-related detraining, where the patient actually regresses – particularly in relation to mobility and functional abilities (Wade 2004).

If the home circumstances of patients with complex care needs are not assessed prior to discharge, to make a 'social diagnosis', it is difficult to evaluate need accurately (Skeet 1970, Amos 1973, Bowling & Betts 1984, McKenna *et al.* 2000). This is significant since these patients are likely to need a greater level of care following discharge than they did before (Bowling & Betts 1984, Victor & Vetting 1988).

The involvement of patients in collaborative goal planning remains problematic, and this impedes opportunities to negotiate appropriate outcomes with the patient (Clark & Dyer 1998, Tripp & Caan 1999). Victor *et al.* (1993) found that patients and their carers remained peripheral to the transfer/discharge process, as did Tripp and Caan (1999), while Waterworth and Luker (1990) found that patients were often reluctant to become involved in decisions about their care.

Person-centred, partnership working, where patient involvement is valued, should be part of the inherent culture of any service caring for clients with complex needs (Wade 2004). This aids agreement in reaching collaborative goals that are meaningful for patients and their discharge care needs, while supporting the value of effective multidisciplinary, inter-disciplinary or trans-disciplinary working (Moroney & Knowles 2006).

Early delays and their impact in the acute sector

Impact of early delays

The pathway of patient care can be greatly enhanced by looking at the processes and systems involved, so as to ensure their timely management and care. Drawing on the principles of the theory of constraints, as described by Shefter (2006), which is, in effect, a systems approach to improvement, has proved helpful throughout different services and settings. By identifying the constraints that hinder patients' progress on their care, strategies to overcome these constraints can be sought – thus reducing length of patient stay.

There are a number of possible reasons for delays at an early stage. With a limited number of therapists and social workers working in the acute sector, priorities need to be decided. In essence, attention is usually given to those who are acutely ill, or those who, with some intervention, can be speedily discharged.

If care is to be transferred to another service, such as intermediate or transitional care, planning for discharge to the final destination is often delayed until the patient reaches this interim setting, as the personnel in the interim setting will be different from those in the acute service. This will delay the commencement of final discharge plans and can lead to a longer overall length of stay than may have been needed. However, there is often quite a time lapse between referral and transfer, which can lead to regression. Any delay at this stage may lead to further delay along the pathway of care, which again may impact upon the well-being and ultimate outcome for the patient and their quality of life. Developing criteria for referral may make this transfer process easier and more efficient (DoH 2003a).

Individuals with complex care needs are also more likely to suffer the vagaries of bed management and moves to other wards. This is because they take longer to recover and because they may need to wait for ongoing care in other settings or services. Once their acute or specialist care needs are resolved, it is these individuals who are most likely to be transferred to make way for new admissions. Moving patients can challenge the ability of staff to remain truly person-centred as they try to get to know the complex care needs of these individuals. Staff may also lose track of care arrangements and progress towards discharge.

Moves can generally be counter-productive, as these patients often have quite specific needs and flourish with staff they know well. Changes can lead to disorientation and regression in individuals with complex needs, even where there is no cognitive impairment (see the case study below, which occurred in 2003).

Case study 1

Case study 1: Rose

Rose had severe arthritis and had been coping at home, with a carer twice a day to help her with personal care and to shop and prepare her meals. She managed quite well with arrangements, using a commode by her chair, which she could just transfer to by herself once up.

One Friday evening, her carer arrived to find her very confused and disorientated. It was late at night, and feeling she could not leave her alone in this state, the carer rang for an ambulance. On admission it became evident that Rose had a urinary tract infection (UTI) and she needed antibiotics, but at this stage she was unable to administer these safely herself. There was no way of accessing intermediate care services at this time so she was admitted to the medical assessment unit (MAU). The next day there was no intermediate care service available to address her needs and she spent 15 hours in bed on the MAU, before being transferred to a medical unit where she remained in bed overnight.

The next day, due to a bed crisis, Rose was identified as a suitable patient to move to a surgical bed and she remained in bed. Rose declined to get up and since rehab was not the focus of the nurses' work on this ward they did not realise how important it was to encourage her to do so. The Monday was a bank holiday so Rose stayed happily in bed. On Tuesday her bed was needed for surgery. As it had not yet been possible to arrange intermediate care, a bed was found back on a medical ward.

By this time Rose was appeared to have a severe infection, and was not well enough for intermediate care. She was also beginning to develop a pressure sore, despite efforts to prevent this. She was now unable to weight-bear and had been found to have Type 2 diabetes so she needed to stay in for further assessment. She was placed on the referral list for the elderly care rehab ward in the acute hospital, but there was no bed.

After two months and several episodes of deterioration, including falling, and several bed moves, a bed became available in the rehab ward and Rose was transferred. By this time she had deteriorated in many ways – including cognition. And it now seemed that the main consideration was whether she needed residential or nursing care!

Mechanisms for timely care and transfer of care

Mechanisms for care

It is evident that acute services need to have in place a mechanism for ensuring that the needs of patients are anticipated and planned for. If this mechanism is in place, referral and transfer of care can occur as soon as it is appropriate and possible. This concept of anticipation may be quite a challenge for team members, especially nurses or junior doctors, who are preoccupied with giving acute or emergency care.

With recent bed and capacity problems, the imperative to move patients on has helped to stimulate the introduction of strategies such as morning consultant ward rounds, progress chasers and tracking teams. The introduction of Gerontology Multidisciplinary Out-reach Teams, from specialist services, with which peer trust is established, can also help immensely (Harwood *et al.* 2002, Robinson & Street 2004). These staff can assess the probable trajectory of care needs of many complex discharge and transfer patients, and make appropriate referrals and arrangements at an early stage. This enables patients to be accepted without further assessment or delay as soon as they are ready and able to be moved. It is often nurses who lead or coordinate these out-reach teams (though not exclusively), as their more generic skills enable them to assess and request referral to other appropriate practitioners such as the occupational therapist, physiotherapist, consultant or geriatrician.

Principles underpinning the process of discharge planning

Underpinning principles

Effective discharge places the individual at the centre of the discharge process. It should promote continuity of care through adequate information and communication flow between patients, carers and services to ensure optimum outcomes for individuals (McKenna *et al.* 2000). Booth and Davies (1991) emphasise that discharge planning is very much a process, rather than a single event. Armitage (1981, p. 386) regarded discharge as: 'a stage in the patient's care which has both a period of preparation and from which there are consequences – it cannot be examined in isolation from what has gone before or separated from what follows after the event when the patient leaves the hospital.'

This concept of discharge is as relevant today as it was in 1981. It can also be linked to the concept of successful aftercare, which can be regarded as 'counteracting or making good any deficiencies in an individual's ability to care for themselves' (New South Wales Health Department 2001).

Victor *et al.* (1993, p.1297) argue that those with complex care needs 'can be very vulnerable to dislocations in the continuous patterns of care provision'. When carrying out effective transfer/discharge there is often a need for a number of different agencies to work together to provide ongoing care for an individual. This may challenge the provision of seamless care (Waters 1987, McKenna *et al.* 2000).

Traditionally, healthcare and social care systems have worked in parallel rather than cooperating with each other. Collaboration has been problematic, and official attempts to make reforms have met with resistance (Glasby & Littlechild 2000, Glasby 2004). This government has prioritised efforts to bring down this 'Berlin Wall' (DoH 2002a, DoH 2006). A range of initiatives and reforms has resulted, although tensions and differences between the healthcare and social care services remain difficult to overcome (Hudson 2000, Glasby 2004).

These initiatives have included the development of a range of strategies such as the Single Assessment Process (DoH2002a, DoH 2002b), and the introduction of a range of intermediate care services, pooled budgets and integrated equipment (DoH 2001, DoH 2003a). More recently, there have been efforts to address the management of long-term conditions and diseases more effectively, with a particular emphasis on the role of community matrons (Sargent & Boaden 2006). Preventative care by GPs, through their Quality of Outcomes Framework (QOF), has also become a central target (DoH 2003b). Finally, it is hoped that the proposed redesign of Primary Care Trusts (PCTs) so that their borders are shared with social services, making them coterminous, will help. Nevertheless, it is recognised that much more still needs to be done to bridge gaps, so although reforms have started there is still a long way to go (DoH 2006).

The process of transfer/discharge planning

The planning process

Staff involved in planning the discharge of those with complex care needs require appropriate skills (McKenna *et al.* 2000). The importance of these skills is often under-estimated and, as Lees and Emmerson (2006) acknowledge, they are often not addressed in pre-registration education. This means that staff members are dependent on learning 'on the job' which, as Weick and Quinn (1999) describe, can be episodic and infrequent. Lees and Emmerson (2006) also found that many staff regarded discharge planning as 'the least interesting and dynamic aspect of their role'.

It is hard to understand how the challenges of complex discharge could be seen as uninteresting (McKenna *et al.* 2000). But personal experience has shown that the constant demands of providing for patients' immediate care needs often push discharge arrangements down to a lower priority, despite their vital importance. As Johnson (1989) suggests, the value of discharge planning is not always recognised by nurses. The degree of importance given to discharge preparation also differs significantly between nurses and their patients, with the latter holding it in higher esteem.

Staff need to develop a comprehensive understanding of the processes involved in planning and preparing for transfer or discharge of care (McKenna *et al.* 2000). This process can be effectively displayed diagrammatically as a flow chart (see page 126), and Jewell (1993) provides a useful example of this, which has been adapted here.

A key tenet of discharge planning is that it should start at or shortly after admission. An expected date of discharge should also be established on admission, or in the case of complex care needs within 24 to 48 hours, during initial assessment (Lees & Holmes 2005). While this has become the gold standard, it has little value unless plans are progressed. In particular, ongoing care needs to be instigated at an early stage (McKenna *et al.* 2000). Some key underlying principles that staff need to follow for successful discharge planning are listed in the table below.

Key principles

Key principles for successful discharge planning
• It should begin as soon as possible.
• Patients and carers should be at the centre of planning, with a clear picture of the outcome they hope to achieve – and any challenges identified.
• There should be comprehensive assessment and documentation.
• Overall multidisciplinary goals should be identified.
• Each discipline should be clear about their input, the intervention, and the time required for these goals to be achieved. A predicted date of discharge based on these should be agreed.
• A named member of the multidisciplinary team should take responsibility for coordinating discharge planning (Annells 2004).
• Any barriers to achieving the goals should be clearly identified and reported, as appropriate, to assist with making good any shortfall.
• Where transfers to other settings are envisaged, planning and arrangements should not be delayed.
• There needs to be effective coordination and constant review and modification, where there is a change in circumstances. This should include a reporting system to ensure that any difficulties are noted and responsibility for acting on these is allocated.
• There must be written discharge procedures.
• Where appropriate, written information should be provided about lifestyle, medication, diet and medical symptoms, etc.
(Adapted from Booth & Waters 1991)

Promoting effective discharge in practice

Teamwork and communication

Effective practice

Effective communication and coordination are essential to expedite efficient discharge planning, although this may not be easy to achieve (McKenna *et al.* 2000, Wade 2004, Moroney &

Clinical practice considerations

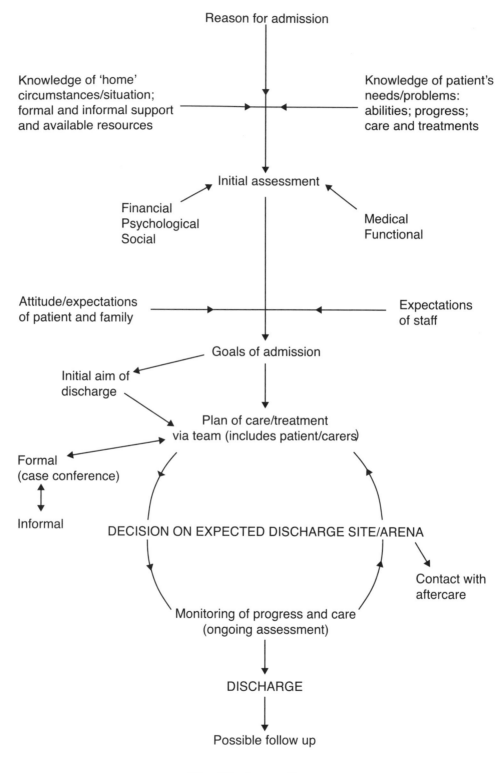

The Discharge Process

Knowles 2006). Similarly, effective teamwork, involving assessment, and anticipatory, holistic, multi-agency working and communication, is vital in order to achieve satisfactory discharge of those with complex needs.

Numerous studies have highlighted the inadequacies of existing processes to ensure accurate, effective recording and transfer of information, along with coordination of activities, both within the service and at the interface with the community. Skeet (1970) found that there was a distinct lack of communication between multidisciplinary teams and patients regarding discharge. This was in 1970, and yet subsequent studies have found that these issues are still causing concern (Patton 1980, DoH 1989 circular (HC(89)5), Victor & Vetting 1988, Curran 1992, Victor et al. 1993, Jewell 1993, Bull & Kane 1996, Tripp & Caan 1999, Werrett et al. 2001, Payne et al. 2002).

Coordination, responsibility and monitoring progress

As we have seen, coordination is pivotal to achieving successful discharge planning and outcomes (Payne et al. 2002). While a multi-skilled and multi-agency approach is essential, as discussed, the importance of the nurse's role in this process should not be under-estimated. Lyon (2006) identifies the nurse as the 'star of the show' in this respect, arguing that nurses can listen and talk to people in a way they understand, and that the nurse is often the only person with any common sense! Nurses are also present over the whole 24-hour period. Likewise, Wade (2004) argues that nurses have the skills and attributes to assess holistically and refer on to specialist services when specific needs are identified, along with excellent skills of coordination (though these are often unrecognised and unsung).

Traditionally, it has been either the consultant or the GP who has taken the final responsibility for discharge from a formal care setting. In rehabilitation and non-acute settings, nurses have probably always tended to see themselves as key to the process, although they have had to inform the doctor as a formality, to obtain tablets to take home (TTOs) and to get discharge letters, where needed. Increasingly, in these contexts and in nurse-led settings the full responsibility is being delegated to nurses, once any medical problems have been resolved. However, nurses still need to have the necessary infrastructure, in terms of the managerial authority to make these decisions, along with the resources to implement them (Werrett *et al.* 2001).

There are a number of organisational activities that provide ways of monitoring and reviewing progress and plans for discharge. These are:

1. The organisation of care in the setting/ward
2. Effective and easily accessible records
3. Well-managed handovers
4. Well-run ward rounds
5. Multidisciplinary discharge planning meetings

The organisation of care in the setting/ward

Whichever method is used, it is essential to ensure that continuity of care is achieved in the best possible way. This is not always easy in the modern NHS where many services have to be available 24 hours a day, 7 days a week, and where there are part-time workers and family-friendly employment policies. Continuity helps staff get to know the complex needs of individual patients and to understand and appreciate subtle changes, or comments they might make, that could otherwise go unnoticed. Staff can also get to know the best way for care to be given, and develop an understanding of some of the behaviour or communication difficulties that the patient may have.

Patients also benefit from this familiarity and are more likely to build up a relationship of trust with staff they know, sometimes disclosing important information related to their care or discharge needs at a time when they feel comfortable and confident about doing so. In this context, however, it is important to be clear about who is responsible for the patient and ensure that information is recorded and highlighted to this person. Care also needs to be reviewed and discharge plans progressed; and these vital elements are often omitted (regardless of the model of care being followed).

Effective and easily accessible records

Collaborative, multidisciplinary records maximise effective communication, as they help to save time, and avoid repetition, gaps in information and discrepancies (Hunt 1999). Somewhere in a very prominent position, at the front of care documentation, must be a place to enter the expected date of discharge, which of course can be changed.

It is also important to have a designated area to document discharge records. This is not just about tick boxes, but must include free text multidisciplinary pages where conversations with patients, family and anyone else involved in the plans can be recorded. This can include discussions at handover, multidisciplinary meetings and case conferences, and any health professional or designated person.

It is vital to document any conversations with patients and their carers if their views and concerns are to be reflected in planning for the future, and to avoid difficulties at a later stage. However, lack of time to document everything contemporaneously is often cited as a reason for not doing this. These records must be maintained, and must also be timely and monitored to account for events during time off. This supports the Single Assessment and represents a more integrated approach to healthcare and social care records (DoH 2006). However, there are several challenges to the effective exchange of information. These include:

- Failure to always share documentation
- Lack of adequate information technology, as identified by nurses in a study carried out by Werrett *et al.* (2001)
- Lack of compatible information technology infrastructure across agencies and Trusts
- Nurses' lack of ability to use and access information technology systems

Well-managed handovers

The handover is often the most mismanaged activity in a service or ward, and yet it can be pivotal to the care and progress of patients (Sexton *et al.* 2004). It is important that the handover is taken seriously and is managed in such a way that time is not wasted, and it does not become disjointed or laborious. Managing handovers is not easy when the needs of staff (e.g. meal breaks, meetings, teaching sessions, supervision, etc.) also have to be considered.

It is not possible to dictate exactly how all services should manage their handovers because each service has to choose the method that seems to work best for them. Taped handovers, bedside handovers, team handovers and team leader handovers are just some of the approaches that may be adopted (Sexton *et al.*

Clinical practice considerations

2004). Meanwhile, some settings suggest that staff read the care notes (though this does depend on having comprehensive records) or provide written handover reports (although here there is a risk of duplicating information). If possible, there should be an opportunity to have a face-to-face discussion about any issues or concerns with a staff member if still on duty.

The table below outlines the information required in the handover report. Following a checklist like this should ensure that time is used effectively to gain appropriate information.

Handover report

Guidance on the information required in a handover report
• Name of patient and location in the ward (the patient must be referred to by name, not be referred to as a bed number)
• Resuscitation status and review date
• Reason for admission and current reason for being here and remaining
• Outline of care needs and brief intervention given (including general and psychological well-being, especially any concerns or anxieties of the patient)
• Any potential risks, e.g. falls, pressure sores, moving and handling, infection, etc.
• Evaluation of progress/lack of progress being made and discussion around any perceived staff/patient concerns
• Any discussions with relatives/carers
• Discussion with multidisciplinary team members
• Discussion/information about medication, including medicines administered, withheld or refused during the shift (if appropriate)
• Planned discharge date and progress of discharge plans/transfer of care plans (any concerns, who needs to be made aware of these, and who will inform them)
• Any outstanding care needs for the oncoming staff
• Any anticipated investigations patient may be receiving during shift or near future, and need for escort or not
Much of this information should form the basis of the care evaluation and any changes in intervention must be recorded and new needs/goals drawn up if appropriate.

Well-run ward rounds

Within medical settings, ward rounds are another important activity. They should always include, as key elements: reviewing/confirming the expected discharge date, interventions still needed, social circumstances, and progress with discharge (Lees *et al.* 2006). It is important for the ward round to involve a nurse who is looking after the patient and knows them as well as possible. This may well mean running ward rounds by teams, so that nurses can change as their team of patients are seen. It may be a bit inconvenient for the doctors, but having a key person present is surely more important.

There needs to be a way of recording information efficiently. This can be done in the medical notes, providing they are sufficiently detailed. Alternatively, some areas use labels with specific information or management plans (Lees *et al.* 2006) recorded during the ward round. An example is shown below (adapted from Moroney & Knowles 2006). Responsibility must be allocated wherever there are actions that need to be undertaken, and the coordinator of care must ensure that the actions are reviewed.

Multidisciplinary team ward round   **Date**.................. **Time**.............

Ward . . . .

Exam

1) Feedback from patient . . . .

2) Feedback from patient's nurse . . . .

3) Review of observations . . . .

4) Evaluation of findings . . . .

Clinical practice considerations

5) Review of prescription and nutritional status . . . .

6) Observation and perceptions of patient . . . .

Plan including:-

Update of bed board . . . .

Referrals . . . .

Investigations:

Nursing interventions and likely time required . . . .

Interventions by therapists and likely timescale

    Physio . . . .

    Occupational Therapists . . . .

    Speech and Language . . . .

    Other . . . .

    Other . . . .

Agreement to refer to . . . .

Social care needs and timescale . . . .

Date referred to Social Services . . . .

Equipment needs and timescale . . . .

Predicted date of discharge . . . .

Any other issues or concerns arising . . . .

. . . .

Multidisciplinary discharge planning meetings

In settings or services where individuals have complex care needs, it is vital to hold multidisciplinary discharge planning meetings. Again, however, it is essential that these are conducted in an effective manner.

It is often difficult to find a time when all the team members are able to attend, due to other care duties/clinics/meetings etc. If a key member is not able to attend, this can sometimes interfere with ongoing plans unless the person has provided adequate details of their progress and concerns. However, Moroney and Knowles (2006) argue that it is still better to go ahead with the meeting.

A good time for many team members may not be a good time for nursing staff to attend, and yet the nurses are key members and central to coordination. Also if a meeting is held at the end of the day, especially at the end of the week, this may make it harder to progress actions. None of these concerns is insurmountable and indeed they are an inevitable part of clinical life. They just show the importance of having a system in place to ensure that careful records are kept of progress and actions that need to be taken.

While focusing on acute care, Lees *et al.* (2006) identified similar difficulties on an emergency admissions ward. They devised a label, similar to the one used for multidisciplinary ward rounds (see pp. 131–132), to provide information that could easily be shared with other colleagues who were not present. This helps to ensure that care is progressed as agreed at the meeting. It may be appropriate to devise a similar type of form to reflect the requirements of those patients with complex needs and their particular setting.

What to cover in a multidisciplinary discharge planning meeting

- First, the purpose of the meeting and expectations of what needs to be achieved should be made clear.
- For each patient presented, there needs to be agreement about:
  - The expected outcome (e.g. where and what level of care)
  - The overall goal and individual goals and plan of care (to achieve the goals) from each member involved
  - The expected/predicted date of discharge, or goals to be

achieved before discharge is agreed so as to estimate predicted date of discharge

- What actions need to be undertaken to achieve discharge on this date, highlighting any significant blocks
- Who is, or needs to be, involved in this

- Each discipline should be clear about what needs to be achieved from their perspective if this outcome is to be achieved.
- Where there are barriers or constraints:
  - These need to be identified and recorded
  - Discussion should take place about what can be done to overcome them and how
  - Individual needs to be identified and responsibility taken for addressing and resolving these, with a date by which it is expected that each one should be resolved
  - The name of the person responsible for each action should be recorded, with a requirement to ensure that feedback is given on progress at the next meeting or sooner, as appropriate
  - If no immediate solution can be found, the appropriate person to inform about this needs to be identified (e.g. the Director of Operations, Social Services or Chief Executive) and someone charged to undertake this, as action may be required at a higher level

Case conferences

Case conferences

If a case is very complex it may be necessary to set up a case conference. This will require the presence of key people, including, where appropriate and possible, the patient. Again, the purpose of such a meeting needs to be made clear and it needs to be well chaired. Past experience suggests that nurses are unwilling to take on this role. Yet they have the skills to chair these meetings, and they are often best placed to do so. The outcomes of case conferences must be carefully recorded, as they address complex issues. They also provide a useful audit trail, and enable individual responsibility to be apportioned. An identified action plan, with a timescale for each aspect, is equally crucial.

Important considerations affecting complex discharges

Complex discharges

Illness trajectory/pathway and timescale

As discussed earlier, for goals to be set and a predicted date of discharge established, a good understanding is needed of the pathway of care, the trajectory and likely timescale of an individual's illness, and the anticipated length of time they will require medical care in hospital. This may not be so easy for those who are frail and have complex needs, as their condition may fluctuate and they may be vulnerable to additional problems when unwell and/or have multiple needs. However, practitioners experienced in the field often have a general timescale in mind. This should act as a starting point, before identifying any constraints envisaged in arranging discharge or where intensive care needs are anticipated.

Risk assessments

Risk assessment will be high on the agenda when making decisions about patients with complex care needs who are going back to their own homes. It is always necessary to undertake appropriate risk assessments, and in some situations it may involve taking some risk, with the possibility that the discharge may not be successful (Wade 2004). While the individual has rights in terms of taking risks for themselves, these cannot be considered in isolation, for their own risks may impose risks on others. For example, a cooking pan accidentally catching fire in the kitchen may well create danger for others if the person is living in shared accommodation such as sheltered housing.

Practitioners need to take many important decisions in relation to risk-taking within rehabilitation and intermediate care services. Risk-taking is 'part and parcel' of successful rehabilitation and needs to be accepted and addressed in a recognised way that forms part of the clinical governance agenda. The decisions related to risk-taking are in addition to the many other decisions that often need to be made, and their importance should not be under-estimated. However, practitioners are perhaps becoming more risk averse because of fear of litigation. Risk aversion on the part of practitioners can have the effect of increasing length of patient

Clinical practice considerations

stay, especially as patients and the public become more aware of what they perceive as their rights and become more litigious, even if this is not always in their best interests.

Similarly, where others are providing care or support, their safety must be considered, and again a risk assessment may be required (Campbell 2001). Psychological risks also need to be considered, for example where a relative is required, or is offering, to give extensive help and has little or no support and little or no relief (not uncommon in contemporary healthcare and social care scenarios). It is important to remember that all carers are eligible for their own carer's assessment (Carers (Recognition of Services) Act, 2000) and to have any benefits clarified and followed up.

Home visits – pros and cons

Waiting for home visits can be problematic, especially as their effectiveness has been questioned (Bore 1994). Clark and Dyer (1998, p. 38) contend that such visits only provide a 'snapshot in time' where safety is usually a priority, and when the patient is often in a state of anxiety. Clark and Dyer go on to discuss how the episodic nature of home visits means that the occupational therapist has little opportunity to monitor or evaluate them.

For these reasons, patients often find themselves with equipment they can't use, don't need or won't use. They may recognise that they need additional or alternative interventions, but don't know who to turn to for help to access them. The recent development of community rehabilitation teams and other intermediate care services may go some way towards resolving these concerns, but as yet there is no parity or consistency in the provision of these services.

Another challenge related to home visits occurs when there is pressure on hospital beds and a home visit may not be managed as well as it could be. In such cases, a hospital discharge may be driven rather by the pressure to empty beds (Means & Smith 1994, Wistow 1995) than being the best way of meeting the patient's needs.

Some areas have established criteria that need to be met to justify a home visit. But whatever the situation, when a home visit is deemed necessary it needs to be timely and to be arranged in a way that does not delay the progress of discharge. In relation to the nurse's role, inappropriate referral for home assessment can certainly delay discharge proceedings, and misdirect resources.

Time may also be spent waiting for therapists to carry out assessments because it is (wrongly) thought that they are the only ones who can conduct such assessments (e.g. washing and dressing).

A home to go to?

Major delays in discharge can occur when a patient is homeless, becomes homeless, or needs adaptations to their home as a result of their changing care needs. In the past, there seemed to be only limited cooperation between health and housing services. This does seem to have improved in recent years, although there are still problems. There is often a need for considerable financial assessment, along with needs assessment. When re-housing is required there may be long delays before appropriate housing become available. And if there are care needs it may not be possible to set up care arrangements until the locality is known, causing further delay. When adaptations are required, there are often issues concerning who owns the property, and there may be delays in getting planning permission before work can even start.

All these challenges point to the importance of the nurse's role in clarifying the situation as early as possible. Plans can then be made, and the availability of a range of transitional care facilities to meet varying levels of need and dependency can be investigated. Failure to plan ahead in this way will often result in days being wasted by inappropriate referrals. In addition, the patient may run health risks associated with delayed discharge, as discussed earlier.

Partnership working

While plans for discharge continue, care needs to be constantly evaluated and revised. It is important to communicate with the individual patient as far as they are able, as well as their family and friends, and any professionals and organisations involved in their care, to try to ensure that anything untoward has been anticipated and that plans seem acceptable (Johnson *et al.* 2003).

As discussed earlier, those with complex care needs may not be able to live independently in the community without help and support from others. The required support needs to be discussed and planned with those who will provide it, while also respecting and involving the patient. In this way, any concerns can be aired at an early stage and taken into account in planning. This should

Clinical practice considerations

increase the likelihood of constraints being overcome by the time the patient is ready to go home. The time spent on interventions to address these constraints is time very well spent. It may also involve accessing certain funding resources, which can take time (see the case study below).

Case study 2

Case study 2: Joe

Joe was a 78-year-old man who lived fairly independently in an upstairs flat. He sustained a stroke and it was evident at a fairly early stage that this would leave some significant left-sided weakness. This was likely to impede his mobility and almost certainly challenge his ability to climb stairs.

Joe was adamant that he wished to return home and so it was essential that plans were instigated at an early stage to discuss the various alternatives to enable Joe to fulfil his wishes. It was clear from the beginning that Joe would probably have residual disability and that changes would be necessary to adapt his flat.

It is true that, at this stage, the full impact of Joe's needs was not yet clear. Nevertheless, acknowledging the likely issues and being open and honest with Joe was important so that plans could be set in motion.

Social care versus healthcare

Social care v healthcare

An acknowledgement of changing population structures and needs, along with a redefining of what constitutes health, led to the introduction of 'The NHS and Community Care Act' (DoH 1990). As a result, more of the needs of those with complex care require-ments are now met by social care as opposed to healthcare. This has left some people feeling deceived by the system, as they believed that the health service would serve them 'from the cradle to the grave'. Many feel very aggrieved when they discover that care that they regarded as 'health' is classified as 'social' and that they are therefore means-tested and required to contribute to funding it. As a result, they feel they have been misled and let down. Some are simply unable to comprehend these changes. And every community has some members who defend their right to healthcare at all costs, for example refusing to be discharged or making sure that they need to return to hospital (see the case study below).

Case study 3

Case study 3: Connie

Connie is a remarkable lady who has a severe kyphosis, rendering her almost doubled over when she walks. Connie owns her own home and has three visits a day to assist her to get up and go to bed, with personal care, and to ensure that she has adequate meals. In fact, despite the difficulties presented by her physical posture, she can actually do much of this herself.

Connie believes that her care needs are health needs. Furthermore, she believes that people like her need to be in hospital. She regularly calls the emergency services, claiming to have fallen, and often manages to get taken in. She has spent extensive time in the intermediate care services and has also been placed temporarily in a care home, which she likes but will not stay in because she has to pay.

Staff members have spent many hours patiently trying to help Connie appreciate that she can manage at home, although she is clearly lonely. She has a daughter who has never been seen by staff, but Connie is not prepared to spend her money on herself and go into care. She believes she has already paid for 'cradle to grave care'.

Further strategies that may enhance discharge planning and outcomes

Further strategies

Drawing upon the theory of constraints

The theory of constraints (as discussed on p. 119) provides one way of addressing some of the constraints identified in discharge planning. The Jonah system is based on this theory, and it has been adopted in the UK. To work at its best, Jonah involves a computerised traffic light system, under which every patient in a caseload is listed.

The various multidisciplinary team members identify goals that the patient needs to achieve before they can reach their destination. This includes any equipment and services that will be required. By recording the estimated time required to achieve the goals, and that required to obtain equipment or set up services, the estimated date of discharge can be agreed. The identified timescale is then divided into green, amber and red. As time passes, the situation may move from green through to red, with green being a 'safe' zone and red indicating danger with regard to exceeding planned length of stay and predicted date of discharge.

Thus the patient will start in green when they are well within the planned timescale for their predicted date of discharge. They may then move into amber, which acts as a warning signal that they are moving towards the date when they should be discharged. If they enter red they have already exceeded, or almost exceeded, the planned date of discharge, and are either at risk of exceeding, or have already exceeded, the anticipated length of stay. Thus moving from green to red provides an alarm system and is meant to trigger more concerted action to progress plans, or highlight the need to explore the constraints or barriers that are causing the delays. If there are evident constraints or barriers further action may be needed, perhaps involving help at a higher level to try to resolve the problems. For instance, if a special chair or bed is needed it may be sourced more easily with the aid of someone in authority who has access to special funding.

Staff members are expected to review progress daily. When it looks as if delays are going to occur, action can be taken to avoid the patient going beyond the original discharge date. When delays do occur, the team members need to find out why. This approach will not solve the problems or constraints. However, it does provide a very structured way of monitoring progress and a means for managers to see what is happening, to ask for explanations, and to try to find ways to overcome the constraints.

For this type of system to work effectively, nurses need to become familiar with it and competent in using it to meet patients' needs and expedite their discharge. In some areas, projects have been established so that staff can become proficient in the use of such a system. The Jonah system, for instance, cannot be used without a commissioned training by the Goldratt company.

Introducing discharge liaison nurses

In many services the introduction or growth of discharge liaison nurses has emphasised the importance of progress in effective discharging (Dinsdale 2002). In some ways it seems a shame that this service is needed, as it could lead to ward staff losing their discharge skills. The advantages, however, are that these specialist staff can develop expertise concerning the services available and establish good working relationships with partnership agencies and parties. They can also help to provide some continuity of care for patients who are moved during a bed crisis. In addition, because the focus of their work is solely on discharge they can spend all their time on this activity, especially when there are time-consuming and complex issues to address. Dealing with this type of complex discharge would really challenge ward staff who are trying to meet a multitude of needs for patients on the wards with minimal staffing levels.

Appointing community matrons

As mentioned earlier, the UK has begun to introduce models of care designed to improve the management of patients with chronic conditions and illnesses. Originally derived from the Evercare model in the USA, the overarching purpose is to optimise the health and well-being of ageing, vulnerable and chronically ill individuals (DoH 2005a).

At the heart of the clinical delivery model is a personal care manager or nurse practitioner known as the community matron. The community matron helps individuals with complex needs to manage their conditions, and any impending crises, with a view to preventing admission where possible. At this point, the evidence is still quite limited in terms of success in reducing bed use. However, these matrons can work very effectively with staff in other services. For instance, if a patient on their caseload is admitted, they can visit and work with the hospital staff to expedite the timely discharge of the patient.

Improving training

As previously mentioned, the education and preparation of practitioners to manage and coordinate complex discharges may sometimes be questionable. Since this is such a key element of the holistic and person-centred care of these individuals, it is imperative that staff members grasp the principles and develop quite sophisticated discharge skills. As Lees (2004, p. 31) points out, it is important that 'nurses have the prerequisite knowledge and skills before adjusting, extending or advancing discharge practice'. The introduction of the 'Agenda for Change' and the 'Knowledge and Skills Framework' provided the ideal means by which this could be achieved, through the introduction of a framework of competencies for staff working with individuals with complex care needs, as has occurred in some settings (Lees 2004, 2006).

Conclusion

Effective and timely discharge of individuals is clearly important if their quality of life is to be promoted and if effective use of resources is to be maximised. Achieving this for those who are frail or who have complex and often fluctuating care needs is not without its challenges. This is particularly true within the large and unwieldy systems of healthcare and social care services, working alongside private or voluntary agencies. An increased focus on a whole systems approach, on better management of the processes involved, on effective mechanisms and a wider range of services to better address patients' needs, has provided a more robust infrastructure. If managed well, this infrastructure can enhance effective discharges. However, this is not to underestimate the demands made on staff involved in complex discharge, particularly as they often work under excessive and relentless pressure. To meet these challenges, they need to be adequately prepared and experienced in using the skills required to deal with complex discharge.

References

Amos, G. (1973). *Care is Rare*. Liverpool: Age Concern.

Annells, M. (2004). 'Discharge from hospital: crocodile-infested water'. *Journal of Clinical Nursing*, 13, 537–538.

Armitage, S. (1981). 'Negotiating the discharge of medical patients'. *Journal of Advanced Nursing*, 6, 385–389.

Bengston, V.L., Rosenthal, C. & Burton, L.M. (1990). 'Families and Ageing: diversity and heterogeneity', in Binstock, R. & George, L. (eds), *Handbook of Ageing and the Social Sciences* (third edition). New York: Academic Press.

Booth, J. & Davis, C. (1991). 'Happy to be home?' *Professional Nurse* (March), 330–332.

Bore, J. (1994). 'Occupational therapy home visits; a satisfactory service?' *British Journal of Occupational Therapy*, 57 (3), 85–89.

Bowling, A. & Betts, G. (1984). 'Communicating on discharge'. *Nursing Times*, 80 (32), 31–32.

Bull, M.G. & Kane, R.L. (1996). 'Gaps in discharge planning'. *Journal of Applied Gerontology*, 15 (4), 486–500.

Campbell, R. (2001). 'Predictors of caregiver burden over a three-month period following hospitalization of the patient'. PhD dissertation, Digital Dissertations, University of Pennsylvania, PA, USA.

Clark, H. & Dyer, S. (1998). 'Equipped for home from hospital'. *Health Care in Later Life*, 3 (1), 36–45.

CSIP (2004/5). 'Planning for Discharge'. Health and Social Care Change Agent Team. (www.cat.csip.org.uk)

Curran, P. (1992). 'Communication of discharge information for elderly patients in hospital'. *Ulster Medical Journal*, 61, 218–223.

Department of Health (1989). 'Discharge of patients from hospital' (Guidance Booklet accompanying Circular HC (89)5, LAC(89) 7).
London: The Stationery Office.

Department of Health (1990). 'The NHS and Community Care Act'.
London: The Stationery Office.

Department of Health (2000). 'Carers (Recognition and Services) Act'.
London: The Stationery Office.

Clinical practice considerations

Department of Health (2001). 'The National Service Framework for Older People'. London: The Stationery Office.

Department of Health (2002a). HSC 2002/001: LAC (2002) 1. 'Guidance on the Single Assessment Process for Older People (and associated Annexes)' (Jan. 2002). London: The Stationery Office. (www.doh.gov.uk/scg/sap/locimp.htm)

Department of Health (2002b). 'Implementing the NHS Plan'. London: The Stationery Office.

Department of Health (2003a). 'Discharge from hospital: pathway, process and practice'. London: The Stationery Office. (www.doh.gov.uk/jointuni)

Department of Health (2003b). 'New GMS and PMS contract: calculation of aspiration payments for the quality and outcomes framework'. London: The Stationery Office.

Department of Health (2005a). 'Supporting people with long-term conditions: An NHS and social care model to support local innovation and integration'. London: The Stationery Office.

Department of Health (2005b). 'The National Service Framework for Long-term Conditions', London: The Stationery Office.

Department of Health (2006). 'Our health, our say: a new direction for community services'. London: The Stationery Office.

Dinsdale, P. (2002). 'Call for radical overhaul of hospital discharge plans'. *Nursing Standard*, 16, 6.

Ellis, B.W. & Johnson, S. (1997). 'A clinical view of pathways of care in disease management'. *International Journal of Health Care Quality Assurance*, 10 (2), 61–66.

Glasby, J. (2004). 'Planning and preparing for intermediate care' (Chapter 6) in *Intermediate Care of Older People*. London: Whurr Publishers Ltd.

Glasby J. & Littlechild R. (2000). *The Health and Social Care Divide: The Experiences of Older People*. Birmingham: Pepar Publications.

Gould, D. (2002). 'Health-related infection and hand hygiene'. *Nursing Times*, 98 (38), 48–51.

Hainsworth, T. (2005). 'A new model of care for people with long-term conditions'. *Nursing Times*, 101 (3), 27–29.

Harwood, R., Kempson, R., Burke, N. & Morrant, J. (2002). 'Specialist nurses evaluate elderly in-patients referred to a department of geriatric medicine'. *Age and Ageing*, 31, 401–404.

Hudson, B. (2000). 'Inter-agency collaboration: a sceptical view', in Brechin, A., Brown, H. & Eby, M.A. (eds), *Critical Practice in Health and Social Care*. Milton Keynes: Open University Press.

Hunt, M. (1999). 'Multidisciplinary case notes: an audit'. *Professional Nurse*, 14 (10), 701–703.

Illich, I. (1975). *Medical Nemesis*. London: Marion Boyars Ltd.

Jewell, S. (1993). 'Discovery of the discharge process: a study of patients discharged from a care unit for elderly people'. *Journal of Advanced Nursing*, 18, 1288–1296.

Johnson, J. (1989). 'Where's discharge planning on your list?' *Geriatric Nursing*, 10, 148–149.

Lasslett, P. (1989). *A Fresh Map of Life*. London: Weidenfeld & Nicolson.

Lees, L. (2004). 'Making nurse-led discharge work to improve patient care'. *Nursing Times*, 100 (37), 30–32.

Lees, L. & Holmes, K. (2005). 'Estimating a date of discharge at ward level: a pilot study'. *Nursing Standard*, 19 (17), 40–43. (www.nursing-standard.co.uk)

Lees L. & Emmerson, K. (2006). 'Identifying discharge practice training needs'. *Nursing Standard*, 20 (29), 47–51.

Lees, L., Allen, G. & O'Brien, D. (2006). 'Using post-take ward rounds to facilitate simple discharge'. *Nursing Times*, 102 (18), 28–30. (www.nursing-times.net)

Lyon, D. (2006). 'Unique care'. Conference Presentation – Managing Long Term Conditions, London (5 March 2006).

Moroney, N. & Knowles, C. (2006). 'Innovation and teamwork: introducing multidisciplinary team ward rounds'. *Nursing Management*, 13 (1), 28–31.

Middleton, S. & Roberts, A. (2000). *Integrate Care Pathways: A Practical Approach to Implementation*. Oxford: Butterworth-Heinemann.

McKenna, H., Keeny, S., Glenn, A. & Gordon, P. (2000). 'Discharge planning: an exploratory study'. *Journal of Clinical Nursing*, 9, 594–601.

Means, R. & Smith, R. (1994). *Community Care: Policy and Practice*. Basingstoke: Macmillan.

New South Wales Health Department (2001). 'Shared responsibility for patient care between hospitals and the community – an effective discharge policy'. Australia: NSW Health Department.

Clinical practice considerations

Oliver, S. (2006). 'Benefits of patient pathways in rheumatoid arthritis care', *Nursing Times*, 102 (16), 28–31.

Oxford Health Authority and Oxfordshire Social Service (May 2002). 'Oxfordshire acute and community hospitals transfer of care (discharge) inter agency standards'. Oxfordshire: Oxford Health Authority and Oxfordshire Social Service.

Patton, M. (1980). *Qualitative Evaluation Methods*. London: Sage.

Payne, S., Kerr, C., Hawker, S., Hardey, M. & Powell, J. (2002). 'The communication of information about older people between health and social care practitioners'. *Age and Ageing*, 31, 107.

Penhale, B. (1997). 'Towards effective discharge planning'. *Health Care in Later Life*, 2 (1), 46–55.

Robinson, A. & Street, A. (2004). 'Improving networks between acute care and an aged care assessment team'. *Journal of Clinical Nursing*, 13, 486–496.

Sargent, P. & Boaden, R. (2006). 'Implementing the role of the community matron', *Nursing Times*, 102 (13), 23–24.

Sexton, A., Chan, C., Elliot, M., Stuart, J., Jayasuriya, R. & Crookes, P. (2004). 'Nursing handovers: do we really need them?' *Journal of Nursing Management*, 12, 37–42.

Shefter, S.M. (Jan-Feb 2006). 'Workflow technology: the new frontier. How to overcome the barriers and join the future'. *Lippincott's Case Management*. 11 (1), 25–34.

Shepperd, S., Parkes, J., McClaren, J. & Phillips, C. (2002). 'Discharge planning from hospital'. *The Cochrane Database of Systematic Reviews*. Issue 1, CD000313. DOI.

Skeet, M. (1970). 'Home from Hospital'. Dan Mason, Nursing Research Committee, Florence Nightingale Memorial Committee, London, Kings Fund.

Stearns, P.N. (1976). *Old Age in European Society*. New York: Holmes & Meir.

Tripp, I. & Caan, W. (1999) 'Is post-rehabilitation discharge of older people successful?' *British Journal of Therapy and Rehabilitation*, 6 (10), 500–504.

Victor, C. & Vetter, N.J. (1988). 'Preparing the elderly for discharge home: a neglected aspect of care'. *Age and Ageing*, 17, 155–163.

Victor, C.R., Young, E., Hudson, M. & Wallace, P. (1993). 'Whose responsibility is it anyway? Hospital admission and discharge of older people in an inner-London District Health Authority'. *Journal of Advanced Nursing*, 18, 1297–1304.

Wade, S. (2004). *Intermediate Care of Older People*. London: Whurr Publishers Ltd.

Waters, K. (1987). 'Discharge planning: an exploratory examination of the process of discharge on geriatric wards'. *British Journal of General Practice*, 41, 72–75.

Waterworth, S. & Luker, K. (1990). 'Reluctant collaborators: do patients want to be involved in decisions concerning their care?' *Journal of Advanced Nursing*, 15, 971–976.

Weick, K.E. & Quinne, R.E. (1999). 'Organisational change and development', *Annual Review of Psychology*, 50 (1), 361–386.

Werret, J., Helm, R. & Carnell, R. (2001). 'The primary and secondary care interface: the educational needs of nursing staff for the provision of seamless care'. *Journal of Advanced Nursing*, 34 (5), 629–638.

Wistow, G. (1995). 'Aspirations and realities: community care at the crossroads'. *Health and Social Care in the Community*, 3, 227–240.

Chapter 8

Occupational therapists and nurses:
Working in partnership to achieve effective discharge planning

Lorraine Marsh and Jo Brady

This chapter looks at the significance of nurses and occupational therapists working in partnership to achieve seamless discharge planning from an acute hospital setting. It also aims to provide a wider knowledge and understanding of the principles, concepts and applications of occupational therapy. All discharge planning is underpinned by accurate information gathering, good communication, effective liaison, and consideration of more than one professional perspective. These aspects will be demonstrated and supported with case examples to show how a holistic, multi-professional approach can increase confidence and empower the nursing team to conduct nurse-facilitated discharges.

Many of the activities that we all carry out in daily life are so familiar that we take them for granted. For the purposes of this chapter, the authors define 'activities of daily living' as those which are necessary for survival and to support 'mind, body and soul'. They define 'function' as the activity of being occupied mentally and/or physically, which is necessary to existence, but is an activity that may not be consciously recognised, i.e. is often 'taken for granted'. Functional status is the cornerstone for determining how and when a patient is discharged. It is at this point that the occupational therapist and the nursing team need to communicate closely to address any concerns that are influencing discharge planning. By working together, they can achieve a safe and coordinated discharge from hospital.

Clinical practice considerations

What is occupational therapy (OT)?

What is OT, why is it important, how does it work, and what role does it have in supporting nurse-facilitated discharge planning?

The *Concise Oxford Dictionary* defines occupational therapy as a 'mental or physical activity designed to assist recovery from disease or injury' (Allen 1990). This is a simple, easily understood definition, yet it does not convey the true implications and value of occupational therapy. The occupational therapist's role is to help patients gain or regain functional independence in all possible aspects of daily activity.

The World Health Organisation (WHO) defines health as not just the absence of illness, but a state of complete physical, social and mental well-being. In order to reach this state, the WHO's charter states that an individual 'must be able to identify and realise aspirations, to satisfy needs and to change or cope with the environment' (1986, cited in Wilcock 2001, p. 11). It is through being occupied and functional, performing tasks or activities, that this is achieved. Being occupied and functional can take many forms, from basic survival needs to 'self-actualisation' (see Glossary, p. 170; Maslow 1954, cited in Young & Quinn 1992, p. 29).

A person needs to function within their environment. The occupational therapist works collaboratively with individuals in the context of their environment to restore or maintain safety and functional ability. This may be achieved by altering the environment or changing the way the activity is performed, and it is determined by the person's functional and cognitive-perceptual ability as well as by their psycho-social (see Glossary p. 169) circumstances. Hagedorn (2000) describes this intervention as a way of restoring or creating a balance between the abilities of the person, the demands of the task and the demands of the environment.

Whether a simple or complex discharge is being planned, the occupational therapist often acts as the 'hub of the wheel'. Standing with the patient and alongside nurses, occupational therapists have a pivotal role in liaising, networking and coordinating with many and varied personnel. The complexity of the discharge plan depends on the patient's circumstances and discharge planning needs and ultimately dictates the level of involvement of the nurse and occupational therapist.

OTs and nurses; working in partnership

The table below illustrates the range of people with whom a hospital occupational therapist regularly communicates to facilitate discharge (Turner 1996). Inevitably, there is some overlap between disciplines, but in liaising with such a broad range of individuals on behalf of the patient, the occupational therapist and nurses together coordinate and drive forward the discharge plan.

Networking for discharge planning

Patient				
Family Friends Neighbours Carers				
WARD	ALLIED HEALTH PROFESSIONALS	COMMUNITY	RESOURCES	AGENCIES
Medical team – Consultants	**Occupational therapists (OTs)**	Social Service OT	Equipment stores	Cultural, religious or voluntary services, e.g. Royal National Institute for the Blind (RNIB)
Nurses	OT technicians Physiotherapist	Community OT and physiotherapist	Equipment suppliers and manufacturers	
Healthcare assistants	Discharge liaison nurses	GP District nurse	Wheelchair assessment centre	
Ward clerks	Speech and language therapists Dietician Chiropodist Psychologist	Social worker Community psychiatric nurse	Functional assessment centre	Employment services City Housing Dept
	Continuing care nurses Psycho-geriatrician interpreters	Assertive case managers Intermediate care	Specialist assessment teams	
	Social workers – hospital and community	Home care services Residential services Wardens		

(Adapted from Turner *et al.* 1996)

Clinical practice considerations

As long ago as 1929, Mattison (cited in Trombly 1995, p. 10) described occupational therapy as providing 'every opportunity for the coordination of all hospital efforts toward returning the patient to community life and economic usefulness'. This description still accurately conveys the importance and value of the occupational therapist's relationship with nurses, in the facilitation of discharge planning. In other words, no single professional is individually responsible for facilitating discharge; it requires liaison and teamwork.

Liaison between the occupational therapist and the nursing team and medical staff is of major importance in establishing a patient's medical status, their likely prognosis and anticipated length of stay. Equally vital to the success of the discharge planning process is liaison with the patient's significant others, such as family, friends, neighbours and carers, who can make vital contributions towards meeting the patient's needs and wishes (Turner *et al.* 1996).

What are the main principles of OT?

Principles of OT

The breadth, depth and scope of OT make it difficult to express fully its value and place in discharge planning. In order to understand and appreciate the role of OT today, we need to look at its philosophy and principles.

According to OT, activity is a central aspect of human experience and well-being. Consequently, the profession also believes that purposeful and balanced activity can be used as a healing force. For these reasons, OT uses activity both as a means of treatment and as an indication of the outcome of treatment. OT is concerned with the individual's engagement in occupation in its widest sense, from purposeful daily activities through to life roles (College of Occupational Therapy 1995).

The profession believes that every individual is unique and that only when treated as an individual will a person be motivated to take responsibility for themselves and secure an independent fulfilled lifestyle. OT believes that the individual (not the disease) should be the focus of treatment. Occupational therapists therefore adopt a client-focused/client-centred style of treatment planning (College of Occupational Therapy 1995).

OTs and nurses; working in partnership

Turner *et al.* (1996, p. 5) succinctly summarise the philosophy of OT:

- People are individuals of worth and inherently different from one another
- Activity is fundamental to well-being
- Where occupational performance has been interrupted, a person can:
  - through the medium of activity develop the adaptive skills required to restore, maintain or acquire function; and/or
  - modify activity in order to facilitate occupational performance.

The above philosophy enables the occupational therapist to collaborate with the patient, the nursing team and other members of the multidisciplinary team. The development of a close working relationship with the nursing team will help achieve a seamless, safe, successful discharge and reduce the risk of re-admission.

OT philosophy is based on adopting a holistic, person-centred, problem-solving approach that views 'purposeful ... activities as a means of restoring health, function and quality of life' (Hagedorn 2000, p. 6). Such activities are considered 'as necessary as food and drink' (Dunton 1917; Miller & Walker 1993, cited in Hagedorn 2000, p. 6).

A problem-solving approach facilitates personal independence and autonomy, and places the focus of intervention on the individual person. Fundamental to its efficacy is the assessment of functional activity and the evaluation of the outcome using the complex process of activity analysis.

What is activity analysis?

Activity analysis

The activities of daily living have been referred to as people being engaged 'in doing simple things' (Hagedorn 2000, p. 3). That which is 'simple' is explained as 'easily understood or done; presenting no difficulty; consisting of or involving only one element or operation' (Allen 1990). However, performing some activities of daily living requires a very complex interaction of skills and abilities. A fundamental principle of OT is to bridge the gap between dysfunction and function. Achieving this requires an understanding of the inherent qualities of the activity, and the

Clinical practice considerations

ability to restructure the activity so that the patient can accomplish it.

Within the hospital setting, where time and resources are limited, the occupational therapist will use an activity that encompasses a wide range of performance components, yet is familiar and non-threatening, e.g. making a hot drink. As demonstrated by the table below, this most routine of tasks requires a complex interaction of mind and body performance components, and clearly consists of more than one element or operation. Perhaps such activities would be better described as 'commonplace' or 'routine and habitual', because referring to them as 'simple' is to devalue their use, meaning and worth.

Precisely because such activities are routine and commonplace, they are often taken for granted and not consciously acknowledged. However, in addressing these complex performance components, occupational therapists can enable people to overcome limitations which compromise their ability to, for example, wash, dress, cook and generally interact with their environment. The value of routine and commonplace activity becomes recognised and appreciated, when, as a consequence of physical or mental limitations, such activities can no longer be achieved.

A key principle in OT is to be able to identify the skills needed to perform an activity and have a thorough understanding of the activity itself. The patient takes an active role in the treatment process but it is professional knowledge and expertise in applying activity analysis skills that decides whether the outcome is a success or not. In essence, it is a problem-solving exercise.

Activity analysis

Performance area	Activities of daily living – Making a hot drink
Performance task analysis	1 Enter kitchen 2 Assemble necessary items 3 Fill kettle 4 Prepare mug 5 Make drink 6 Drink tea

Performance components

Performance demands (Emboldened terms are explained in the Glossary on p. 169)

Motor	Sensory	Cognitive	Perceptual	Emotional	Social
Mobility	Proprioception	Motivation (thirst)	Visual/tactile – temperature	Gratification	Communication
Standing balance/ tolerance	Coordination – especially hand/eye	Social – knowledge of activity and where it occurs	Figure/ground discrimination		Interaction
Muscle strength					Social skills
Exercise tolerance	Visual/tactile – in unison and separately	Decision making	Form constancy		
		Judgement	Praxis		
Energy levels/oxygen	Degrees of touch, temperature and pressure	Memory and knowledge	Gnosis		
Gross movements of upper body – bending, stretching, reaching – core stability	Body awareness	Logical and sequential thought	Object recognition		
	Sensation of movement	Organisational skills	Depth perception		
Gross movements of upper limbs – shoulder **ab/adduction**, rotation, forearm **pronation/ supination**	Hearing Smell Taste Thirst satisfied	Safety awareness	Appreciation of form and colour		
		Maintaining attention and concentration	Stereognosis		
Fine movements of upper limbs – wrist and hand, grip ability and strength, joint flexion/extension					
Hand-to-mouth coordination					
Sip and swallow					

(Adapted from Turner *et al.* 1996)

Raising awareness of functional performance in activities of daily living to assess the impact of illness and disability, will inform the nursing team when facilitating discharge.

Clinical practice considerations

How can nurses and occupational therapists work in partnership to create tailor-made discharge plans?

Tailor-made plans

Effective discharge planning should be multidisciplinary in nature, timely, proactive and patient-centred. It should take account of key factors such as the patient's usual living arrangements, and ensure that the patient's health and functional safety are not compromised after discharge.

In order to support the nurses in facilitating discharge planning, as previously mentioned, the occupational therapist contributes an in-depth assessment. Liaison with the nursing team produces a discharge plan which is tailor-made to meet patient needs, upholding patient autonomy and advocating choice and partnership in the therapeutic process (College of Occupational Therapists 2005). The diagram below illustrates the OT process, highlighting the interaction with the nursing team.

The occupational therapy process

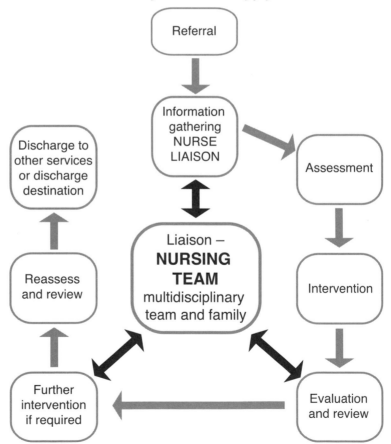

OTs and nurses; working in partnership

The next three diagrams illustrate OT intervention and nurse collaboration in providing 'tailor-made', patient-centred, needs-led discharge planning.

Rapid assessment and discharge

Rapid assessment & discharge

Jean is a 56-year-old woman admitted to hospital with exacerbation of chronic obstructive pulmonary disease (COPD). She lives with her husband, who is employed in the building trade, in a two-storey house. She is independent with personal hygiene but reports not managing well with 'domestic activities of daily living' due to breathlessness and decrease in energy levels.

Referral to discharge (36 hours)

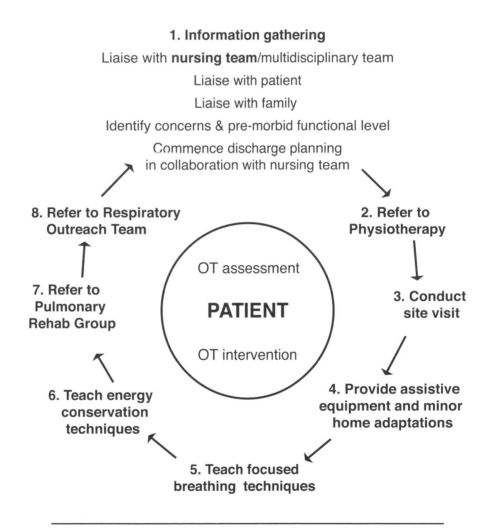

1. Information gathering
Liaise with **nursing team**/multidisciplinary team
Liaise with patient
Liaise with family
Identify concerns & pre-morbid functional level
Commence discharge planning
in collaboration with nursing team

8. Refer to Respiratory Outreach Team

2. Refer to Physiotherapy

OT assessment

PATIENT

OT intervention

7. Refer to Pulmonary Rehab Group

3. Conduct site visit

6. Teach energy conservation techniques

4. Provide assistive equipment and minor home adaptations

5. Teach focused breathing techniques

Clinical practice considerations

Short to medium-term length of stay

Miriam is a 76-year-old woman who has been admitted to hospital with increasing confusion and urinary frequency. She has a past medical history of arthritis, upper respiratory tract infection, multiple urinary tract infections and early-onset dementia. She lives alone in a house, and her family visit regularly and complete shopping calls and heavy housework. Her family have raised concerns about her safety at home.

Referral to discharge (2 weeks)

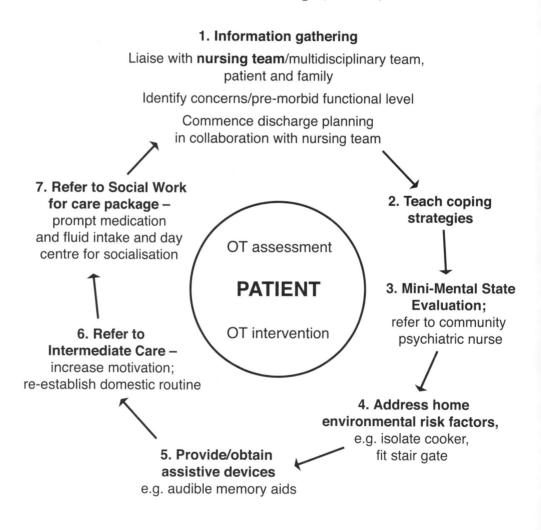

1. Information gathering

Liaise with **nursing team**/multidisciplinary team, patient and family

Identify concerns/pre-morbid functional level

Commence discharge planning in collaboration with nursing team

7. Refer to Social Work for care package – prompt medication and fluid intake and day centre for socialisation

2. Teach coping strategies

OT assessment

PATIENT

OT intervention

3. Mini-Mental State Evaluation; refer to community psychiatric nurse

6. Refer to Intermediate Care – increase motivation; re-establish domestic routine

4. Address home environmental risk factors, e.g. isolate cooker, fit stair gate

5. Provide/obtain assistive devices e.g. audible memory aids

OTs and nurses; working in partnership

In-patient rehabilitation

Peter is a 46-year-old man who has had a below-knee amputation. He lives with his wife in a two-storey house. He is a computer graphics designer.

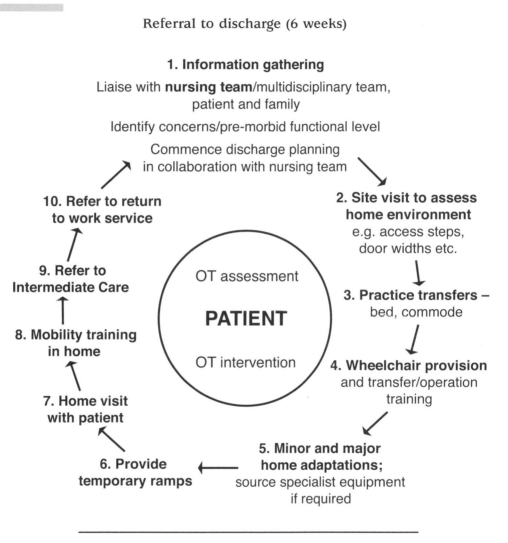

Referral to discharge (6 weeks)

1. Information gathering

Liaise with **nursing team**/multidisciplinary team, patient and family

Identify concerns/pre-morbid functional level

Commence discharge planning in collaboration with nursing team

10. Refer to return to work service

2. Site visit to assess home environment
e.g. access steps, door widths etc.

9. Refer to Intermediate Care

8. Mobility training in home

OT assessment

PATIENT

OT intervention

3. Practice transfers –
bed, commode

4. Wheelchair provision
and transfer/operation training

7. Home visit with patient

6. Provide temporary ramps

5. Minor and major home adaptations;
source specialist equipment if required

Medical, social and functional fitness

Defining medical, social and functional fitness is a complex and multi-dimensional process. These three aspects of fitness are very briefly summarised here, to demonstrate their value and the need to interlink them in the discharge planning process.

Clinical practice considerations

Medical
fitness

Medical fitness

Medical fitness can be described as a pathological state which is represented by deviation from 'normal' parameters of the body. The medical model defines being healthy as the 'absence of disease' and as 'functional fitness'. This concept dates back to the need to produce an efficient workforce during the 1940s (Jones 1994). At this time, being 'not ill' and being able to walk were the minimum criteria for being healthy enough to be called up to serve in the army.

Historically, decisions about health and disease used to be regarded by doctors as matters for them alone. Patients had a passive role. Having been told what was the matter with them (and sometimes not even that), their only task was to obey whatever instructions the doctor thought fit to issue. Most modern definitions of health continue to be based on the notion that when medical symptoms have been addressed or resolved the person is medically fit.

Disease (or 'dis-ease') is a term that evolved from its original meaning of a state of being 'not at ease' to one that describes a biomedical reductionist view of the body. For an occupational therapist, the concept of functional fitness goes far beyond 'an absence of disease'. OT is not solely concerned with the biological and physiological processes of the body. It also encompasses the psychological, environmental and social aspects.

Functional
fitness

Functional fitness

Functional fitness is very important in achieving a successful discharge and can have different meanings in different situations. An occupational therapist deals with the everyday activities that are performed without conscious thought or effort, such as getting in or out of bed, washing your face, or preparing a meal. It is only when these activities cannot be performed that you notice you were doing them at all. They are the 'taken for granted' basic building blocks of everyday living.

For example, a broken arm will significantly compromise your ability to wash, dress, feed yourself or attend to toilet hygiene. Arthritis in knees and hips will compromise mobility. So how does an individual access their kitchen to prepare meals, or reach the only toilet if it is upstairs? Hence, although an individual may be

OTs and nurses; working in partnership

deemed medically fit for discharge they may not be functionally fit. In other words, they may have lost the ability to address personal care or domestic routines.

It has also been found that an individual's perception of their functional fitness is heavily influenced by their 'social status, values and norms, which are also influenced by roles and environmental factors' (Turner *et al.* 1996, p. 104).

Social fitness

Social fitness

Social fitness depends on the patient's perspective, i.e. their way of seeing, knowing and doing, and will be dominated by their cultural and social influences. These societal and cultural influences are also inextricably bound up with, and therefore reinforce different values, motivations and behaviours (Jones 1994).

Social fitness may also depend on other material factors that may be outside an individual's control, e.g. damp housing, poor diet, reduced mobility, or lack of formal/informal care or support. From the social perspective, 'the support of family and other social systems are most important in enhancing the capacity of (patients) to function in their daily lives' (Kielhofner 1992, p. 7).

The multidisciplinary team as a whole generally takes a patient-centred approach to discharge. However, as previously discussed, the occupational therapist is the only member of the team who uses activity analysis to evaluate the impact of illness/disability on function within the patient's normal environment. Working together, with an understanding of each other's perspectives and philosophies, the nursing team and occupational therapist can enhance the patient's experience by achieving timely and appropriate discharge planning.

Two case studies (see below) may help to illustrate the importance of considering all three aspects of fitness – medical, functional and social.

Case Study 1

Case study 1: Mr G.

Mr G., aged 70, lives alone in a house. He was previously independent with mobility, personal and domestic activities of daily living. He has no relatives but a neighbour gets the heavy shopping once a week. Following a collapse at home and being found by his neighbour, Mr G. was admitted to hospital and diagnosed as having experienced a stroke. On admission, Mr G. presented with right side weakness, poor mobility and slurred speech.

Within four days, Mr G. reported to nursing staff that he was washing independently, mobilising independently around the ward and speech was almost back to normal. All medical aspects had been addressed so discharge was planned forthwith. However, a nurse mentioned to the ward OT that she had observed Mr G. wearing his shirt back to front and trying to comb his hair with the tube of toothpaste. Consequently, the nurse requested a full OT assessment.

Following OT assessment, it was determined that although Mr G. had appeared outwardly to regain his previous level of function, it was severely compromised due to his perceptual processing ability being affected. When moved from the ward setting (where demands on functional ability are few) to the OT Assessment Unit, Mr G. was no longer able to perform basic personal care and domestic tasks appropriately and safely. He was unable to recognise items of clothing and how he should dress; he had lost the ability to name objects and know their function; he was unable to sequence a task and tended to perseverate an action (e.g. repeatedly wash his face and nothing else). He also required prompting to initiate and maintain an activity.

All of the above would significantly affect Mr G.'s functional safety at home. Mr G. did, however, demonstrate a capacity to make his own decisions and expressed a wish to return home.

Very close liaison occurred between Mr G., his neighbour, a social worker and the OT to establish an appropriate care package, as well as consultation with Intermediate Care for ongoing rehabilitation at home. Once all plans were established and in place, Mr G. was discharged home.

If Mr G. had been discharged when 'medically fit' there would have been a high risk of an accident occurring, perhaps as a consequence of washing the electric kettle in the sink or switching on the gas cooker and not lighting it. By addressing the medical, functional and social perspectives together, the risk of re-admission was reduced and a safe, successful discharge was achieved.

Case study 2: Mr A.

Mr A., aged 75 and living alone since his wife died four months ago, has been admitted to hospital six times in the last ten weeks with diarrhoea and vomiting. No particular medical cause has been identified. Following resolution of the episode, the patient is discharged home, having only seen medical staff.

A seventh admission occurs nine days later for the same complaint. A nurse, concerned that he may not be coping at home even though he seems physically and functionally independent whilst on the ward, discusses the patient with the ward occupational therapist. Following a thorough OT assessment, it is discovered that the patient's wife used to do all the cooking and shopping; the patient has limited cooking skills and poor awareness of food hygiene; his fridge has not worked properly for the last three months and, for financial and functional reasons, he is not able to buy a new one.

Using clinical reasoning and problem-solving skills, the occupational therapist surmises that the diarrhoea and vomiting are inevitable consequences of eating less than thoroughly cooked food and potentially contaminated food.

OT recommendations:

- A referral to be made to Social Work for financial advice and assistance to purchase a fridge and establish support for shopping.
- The patient to be found a transitional care bed until fridge is purchased.
- A referral made to Intermediate Care for rehab at home to teach food hygiene and cooking skills.

Social and cultural challenges to effective discharge

Clearly, if patients' functional and social needs are not addressed they are likely to be at high risk of re-admission. They may also require more serious and more costly medical intervention as a consequence of potentially avoidable accidents or worsening of medical conditions.

Clinical practice considerations

It is evident that all three perspectives on fitness have key roles to play in the patient's journey from admission to discharge. Failure to recognise or acknowledge the value of complementary approaches can give rise to misunderstanding, miscommunication and conflict. However, cultural, situational and political factors can sometimes exacerbate already difficult situations. Some cultures 'may encourage the maintenance of the sick role and the acceptance of how sick people perform' (Sumsion 1999, p. 35). This can and does lead to 'knee-jerk' responses to relatives' persistent and sometimes unrealistic requests. The resultant pressure can lead to multidisciplinary team communication dissolving, confusion and contradictions arising, and discharges being delayed unnecessarily.

Patients and relatives may also have unrealistic expectations of the hospital experience and anticipated length of stay. We must remember that, for the elderly population, hospital care has changed out of all recognition. For instance, many individuals still use the term 'convalescence' when health professionals are referring to Intermediate Care rehabilitation and getting patients home as soon as possible.

The multidisciplinary team must maintain a balance between professional perspectives, government directives and the realities of discharge planning. The team members must trust and respect each other's professional skills, expertise and judgement.

Clearly, there is a need to be flexible to meet the needs of the patient. The table opposite demonstrates that we must approach discharge planning 'at a level that facilitates the resolution of problems rather than adding to them' (Sumsion 1999, p. 34), to support the patient in achieving a personally acceptable lifestyle within their cultural and social environment. In order to achieve positive discharge outcomes, each multidisciplinary team member needs to communicate proactively and concisely, while recognising the value of partnership and a whole systems approach.

OTs and nurses; working in partnership

Nurses and occupational therapists: Achieving a positive discharge outcome through effective communication.

76-year-old man. Unstable blood sugar levels. Wife and supportive family. Lives in first-floor flat (no lift). Family keen for discharge home. Son states care package being set up by community social worker and family will be assisting patient's wife until services in place. Medics have documented that the patient is medically fit for discharge the next day.

ACTION	OUTCOME
Scenario A Single patient record information taken at face value Transport and Tablets to Take Out (TTOs) arranged Patient discharged home into care of family District nurses informed of discharge	**Scenario A** Next day post-discharge district nurse attended to administer insulin Found patient had slept in chair as wife unable to transfer patient into bed or onto the commode Patient re-admitted to hospital
Scenario B Concerned re: patient transfer status – maximum assistance x 2 to achieve any transfers Patient referred to Physio & OT OT conducted thorough assessment and liaised with multidisciplinary team Social Work dept contacted; advised that patient was not due a review for another 6 months and no existing care package was in place Met with family to gain pre-morbid functional status Required minimal assistance x 1 to transfer Wife provided all care – feeding, personal hygiene Warden-controlled ground-floor flat secured Discussed care package – family agreed to have one morning call per day to assist patient's wife as other family members work full time Social Work referral made Intermediate Care rehab bed agreed to by family on behalf of patient – referral made	**Scenario B** Patient transferred to Intermediate Care Care package established Move to ground-floor flat achieved All functional and social needs addressed Re-admission risk avoided

Clinical practice considerations

The way forward: Supporting nurse-facilitated discharge

The way forward

Discharge planning requires the skills of more than one health professional and is, therefore, a multi-faceted process. It has been defined as the systematic identification and organisation of services and support to assist patients to manage in the community after discharge (Shepperd & Iliffe 2002). This requires nurses, doctors and allied health professionals to understand and interpret patients' and carers' needs, from both the patient's and carer's perspectives.

This approach also assumes that health professionals understand the patient's home environment and the social support available, as well as the patient's ability to regain their previous level of functional ability once they have left hospital. Most importantly, the health professionals need to know whether or not the patient's needs can be met within the community setting.

Discharge planning is a core skill for occupational therapists, and forms part of a formal academic OT programme. However, it is not deemed to be so important for all health professionals. Lees and Emmerson (2006) identified formal discharge planning skills as being absent from the didactic pre-registration nursing education syllabus. Instead, the nurse acquires many discharge skills by learning 'on the job'. This may be viewed in a negative light. However, it must be remembered that there is much value and relevance in experiential learning (or 'learning on the job'). As previously mentioned, every patient requires a tailor-made discharge plan. And producing an effective tailor-made discharge plan often requires experience as much as formal training. So it is through team working, mutual respect and understanding of each other's roles, in conjunction with collaborative planning, that experience will be gained and learning achieved.

From an occupational therapist's perspective, case management includes assessment (of the patient and their environment), evaluation, activity analysis, problem solving and risk management, which are all fundamental core skills (Hagedorn 1997). Using their clinical judgement, expert knowledge of risk assessment and case management skills, occupational therapists are therefore a valuable resource to support nurse-facilitated discharges.

Having reviewed the literature, it has become evident to the authors that an enormous amount has been written about hospital discharge. The Department of Health has produced a number of guidelines, workbooks and initiatives on the subject. These documents have established that, in order to effect a good, safe discharge, planning should begin soon after admission, in the case of emergency or non-planned admission, and at pre-assessment clinics for planned admissions. The patient and their carers should also be involved in the discharge planning process.

What occurs during discharge planning can have a major impact on the patient's experience of being in hospital and their eventual return home. Delays in discharging patients back to their home environment can have a negative effect on long-term outcomes. The results of such delays may include loss of confidence, loss of independence, loss of autonomy and the risk of hospital-acquired infections (House of Commons Health Committee 2002).

Above all, we need to adopt a patient-centred approach, focusing on the needs of individual patients and their carers. The patients and their carers can then play a meaningful role in the discharge process, thereby reducing the risk of re-admission to hospital and, importantly, premature entry into residential care.

Jacqui Smith, Minister of State for Health, in her Foreword to 'Discharge from hospital: pathway, process and practice' (DoH 2003), states that: 'It is increasingly evident that effective hospital discharges can only be achieved when there is good joint working between the NHS, Local Authorities, housing organisations, primary care and the independent and voluntary sectors, in the commissioning and delivery of services including a clear understanding of respective services. Without this, the diverse needs of local communities and individuals cannot be met.'

Conclusion

This chapter has identified the focus of OT and explained how a better understanding of the occupational therapist's role can help the nursing team to further develop their skills in facilitating

Clinical practice considerations

hospital discharges. By pooling resources and emphasising the ethos of cohesive team working, nurses can become valuable mediators. They form a vital link between the patient, the occupational therapist and other health professionals during the discharge planning process.

It must be remembered that a whole systems approach to discharge planning can only be accomplished through partnership working. It is not what we do as individual professionals but how individual professionals do it as a team ('it's not what we do, it's the way that we do it'). Nurses and occupational therapists will achieve this by being allies in the discharge planning process and promoting 'joined-up thinking', the sharing of information, collaborative participation in learning and development training programmes, and above all by demonstrating ownership of, and commitment to, seamless discharge planning.

Glossary

Glossary

abduction A motion that pulls away from the mid-line of the body, e.g. raising the arms laterally to the side.

adduction A motion that pulls towards the mid-line of the body, e.g. dropping the arms to the side.

cognitive-perceptual ability The mental ability to receive, register and process sensory information, resulting in a set of mental operations performed to reach a common functional goal.

core stability The ability to control the position and movement of the core muscles of the torso (spine, pelvis and shoulder), creating a solid base of support for movement of the extremities.

figure-ground discrimination The isolation of a shape or object from its background.

form constancy The ability to recognise two objects which have the same shape but different size or position, e.g. 'b' and 'd', 'p' and 'q', or 'm' and 'w'.

gnosis The ability to recognise objects or faces.

Mini-Mental State Examination (MMSE) The most commonly used test for memory problems or when a diagnosis of dementia is being considered.

praxis The ability to execute intentional movements correctly.

pronation A rotation of the forearm that moves the palm to face down.

proprioception The sensory feedback mechanism for motor control and posture.

psycho-social Referring to the psychological and social influences that determine human behaviour.

Clinical practice considerations

self-actualisation The realisation of an individual's full potential (see Maslow 1954 for detailed explanation).

stereognosis The ability to determine what an object is by using the modality of touch.

supination The opposite of pronation; rotation of the forearm so that the palm faces up.

OTs and nurses; working in partnership

References

Allen, R.E. (1990). *The Concise Oxford Dictionary.* Oxford: Oxford University Press.

American Occupational Therapy Association (1994). 'Uniform Terminology for Occupational Therapy' (3rd edn). *The American Journal of Occupational Therapy,* 48 (11), 1047–1054.

College of Occupational Therapists (2005). 'Code of Ethics and Professional Conduct'. London: College of Occupational Therapists.

Department of Health (2003). 'Discharge from hospital: pathway, process and practice'. London: The Stationery Office.

Hagedorn, R. (1997). *Foundations for Practice in Occupational Therapy.* UK: Churchill Livingstone.

Hagedorn, R. (2000). *Tools for Practice in Occupational Therapy*. UK: Churchill Livingstone.

House of Commons Health Committee (2002). 'Delayed Discharges' (third report of session 2001–2002 HC, CM5645). London: The Stationery Office.

Jones, L.J. (1994). *The Social Context of Health and Health Work*. UK: Palgrave Macmillan.

Kielhofner, G. (1992). *Conceptual Foundations of Occupational Therapy.* Maryland, USA: Williams & Wilkins.

Kielhofner, G. (1995). *A Model of Human Occupation* (2nd edn). Maryland, USA: Williams & Wilkins.

Lees, L. & Emmerson, K. (2006). 'Identifying discharge practice training needs'. *Nursing Standard*, 20 (29), 47–51 (www.nursing-standard.co.uk).

Maslow, A.H. (1954). *Motivation and Personality*. New York: Harper & Row.

Mattison, J.A. (1929). *Occupational Therapy and Rehabilitation* (cited in Trombly 1995, p. 10).

Miller, R.J. & Walker, K.F. (eds) (1993). *Perspectives on Theory for the Practice of Occupational Therapy*. Aspen, USA: Gaithersburg.

Shepperd, S. & Iliffe, S. (2002). 'Hospital at home versus in patient care'. *The Cochrane Library*, 2, 81–82.

Sumsion, T. (ed) (1999). *Client-Centred Practice in Occupational Therapy.* UK: Churchill Livingstone.

Clinical practice considerations

Trombly, C.A. (1995). *Occupational Therapy for Physical Dysfunction* (fourth edition). Maryland, USA: Williams & Wilkins.

Turner, A., Foster, M. & Johnson, S.E. (1996). *Occupational Therapy and Physical Dysfunction* (4th edn). USA: Churchill Livingstone.

Wilcock, A.A. (2001). *Occupation for Health, Vol 1, A Journey from Self Health to Prescription.* UK: British College of Occupational Therapists.

World Health Organisation (1986). 'The Ottawa Charter for Health Promotion'. Canada: Health and Welfare Canada, Canadian Public Health Association.

Young, M.E. & Quinn, E. (1992). *Theories and Principles of Occupational Therapy.* UK: Churchill Livingstone.

Chapter 9

Discharge and medication

Ross Groves

Despite the best efforts of the healthcare professionals and ancillary staff who work in hospitals, the phrase 'you can go home' is often the most welcome news that a patient receives during their time in hospital. A wide range of issues may impact greatly on the patient's life once discharged; not least of these is their medication. This chapter will discuss some of the difficulties faced by patients, nurses and healthcare professionals in understanding why and how medication may change or be introduced during a hospital stay. It will also consider how best to ensure accurate continuation of supply at and after discharge.

Few patients leave hospital without any medication. Surgical and manipulative procedures may require pain relief and/or antibiotics; medical monitoring of a long-term condition may necessitate a change in a patient's drug therapy; or the discovery that a patient is suffering from a previously undiagnosed disease may mean that new drugs will have been initiated. For this reason, the process of managing medicines appropriately for a patient's needs is at the heart of effective discharge planning.

The importance of good communication

Good communication

Various changes have been made in the NHS to provide a pharmacy service that is responsive to patients' needs during their stay in hospital. Yet there is still a need for more effective communication about drug interventions. There are tremendous opportunities for nurses, both hospital and community-based, to expand their practice to collaborate with pharmacists for the benefit of patients. But this cannot happen without good communication between all the many 'partners' involved in the patient's care. Without effective communication, most changes will be counterproductive. On discharge, the first point where communication can, and often does, fragment is between secondary and primary care.

Healthcare professionals should be aware of treatment changes for patients they are responsible for, but the patient is sometimes left out of the loop. If this happens, serious confusion can arise from the patient's lack of knowledge and understanding, both of medication schedules in general and changes to those schedules in particular. Solving this problem is vital, in order to ensure that effective treatments are used both in and out of hospital. Nurses are ideally placed to work with pharmacists, doctors and other prescribers to help the patient get the best from both formally prescribed and informally purchased medication.

Medication at admission, at hospital and at discharge

Medication

It is important to remember that patient discharge from hospital is just one stage in a continuum of care, from home to hospital, and back again. The diagram below shows how an individual might move from their routine life at home to a situation where a medical (or occasionally social) problem arises that necessitates an in-patient stay. If all goes well, the problem can be addressed in hospital and the patient can then return home.

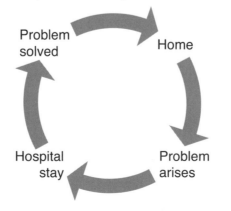

Discharge and medication

Drug treatments are often taken for granted, both by patients and by professionals. The patient may not realise, and the professionals may ignore, the effect that any chemical taken into the body can have. Involving the patient and encouraging them to continue taking responsibility for management of their existing medication whilst in hospital is therefore crucial to achieving timely discharge.

Obtaining a drug history on admission

On admission a full drug history should be obtained. This should include everything that a patient ingests, inhales, injects, inserts or applies. Despite the difficulties encountered in extracting all relevant information from the patient, the record should include:

- Foodstuffs
- Drinks
- Prescribed medication
- Purchased medication
- Smoking
- Illicit drug use
- Herbal remedies
- Alternative therapies

Ideally, all food and drink consumed by a patient should be listed. Many chemicals in foods interact with drugs, quite apart from the effect they have on general health. Alcohol isn't any more important than sugar or caffeine drinks, as far as pharmaceutical effects go. However, in practice, most histories only give a general picture.

All the above items can independently affect the patient's health and may also interact with each other. Such effects can be detrimental but on occasion may be beneficial. Issues that could arise might include:

1. A predominantly fatty diet causing obesity and/or possible changes in absorption and distribution of medication
2. Vegetarian/vegan diet causing lack of specific nutrients such as vitamin B12 and folate (needed for nerve regeneration and cell division)
3. Excessive alcohol/caffeine intake
4. Decreased water consumption
5. Not taking prescribed medication (will they tell you?)
6. Using over-the-counter (OTC) medications that are similar to prescribed medications, e.g. paracetamol preparations

Clinical practice considerations

7. Nicotine having a beneficial effect on concentration, while the tar content of cigarettes causes heart disease
8. Cardiovascular effects of heroin
9. Not mentioning illicit drug use and herbal remedies (e.g. St John's Wort), many of which interact with prescribed medication
10. Absorption of massage/aromatherapy oils through the skin, causing irritation

Who is best placed to elicit this information? The answer may well be a combination of individuals with the appropriate knowledge base to detect potential and actual problems. However, these professionals may not be able to speak to the patient on admission, and the patient's GP, private physician and community pharmacy/pharmacies should be involved. In addition, in cases where patients have been transferred from nursing or residential settings (including interim and intermediate care), the staff from these settings can also play a crucial part in obtaining the drug history. Whoever gets the information, it is important to ensure that as much as possible is found out about how a patient takes their medication. The reality may differ significantly from the intention of the prescriber or from the information given to the patient by the dispensing pharmacist! Such differences may have a significant impact on the patient's health and can, indeed, contribute to admissions.

Here are two examples:

1. Patient admitted to a nursing home who developed digoxin toxicity when given the prescribed dose every day and so needed hospital treatment.
2. Patient's analgesia changed (in accordance with Primary Care Trust (PCT) policy) to co-codamol, which did not relieve their pain. Patient borrowed co-dydramol (their original analgesic) from a neighbour, took both and developed hepatic problems due to paracetamol overdose. This led to re-admission.

Nurse prescribing as part of the admission process

Although some hospitals now employ admission pharmacists who are available to discuss medication with patients on arrival, nurses remain the most frequent point of contact on admission. Since 2002, the advent of supplementary and independent nurse prescribing has increased the number of nurses with more detailed

Nurse prescribing

pharmacological knowledge but these may not always be the nurses who admit the patient. If they were, prescribing on admission would be much simpler. It would no longer be necessary to attempt to contact the doctor or pharmacist on call to transcribe medication to the drug sheet. Medication could be prescribed immediately.

The introduction of nurse-led admission and discharge policies should provide an effective framework for transferring patients into and out of hospitals safely, sensitively and efficiently. Any nurse involved in such an initiative should have the skills, knowledge and experience to ensure that medication and other ongoing care continues appropriately. Nurse prescribers would be ideally placed to carry out such a role.

Using the patient's own medication while in hospital

Patient's own medication

Many hospitals allow the use of Patient's Own Drugs (PODs). These are sometimes called Patient's Own Medications (POMs), or they may have another acronym, specific to that institution. In the past, patients' medication was taken from them on admission and disposed of, causing significant wastage.

Nowadays PODs schemes allow any medication brought into hospital to be kept in a locked cupboard by the patient's bed, provided that there is an acceptable system in place to facilitate this. PODs can then be used during the patient's stay and are also available to be taken home, thus removing the need for a prescription to be dispensed on discharge. Changes in medication during a stay can also be facilitated, more easily than formerly, using this system.

Medication on discharge

Medication on discharge

If communication and education about medication on admission is important, then communication and education about medication on discharge is equally vital, if not more so. All parties involved in the further supply of drug therapies need to know what changes have been made to medication schedules during the patient's stay. They should also know why these changes have been made, so that the correct information can be communicated to the patient.

The drug supply difficulties that may arise on discharge are many and varied. Their significance may be interpreted differently

Clinical practice considerations

by each individual involved, but they can all have a serious impact on the patient's experience of discharge. These are some of the problems that can occur:

- Delays in obtaining take-home medication: irritating for the patient and for hospital bed managers
- Lack of understanding of changes in medication: confusing for patient, carers, GP and pharmacists involved in administration and supply at home
- Delayed communication of new dosage schedules and new drugs to GP practice and community pharmacy responsible for supply: may result in incorrect medication (sometimes the drug regime that was in place before admission) being prescribed and supplied to the patient, thus causing more confusion and potential harm

Having an identified or named nurse responsible for patients' discharge should help to resolve such problems. For example, the nurse will have developed a rapport with the patient during their stay and the patient will have opportunities to discuss their drug therapy. As with admissions, the ability of the nurse to write a take-home prescription or authorise such a supply should also speed up the process (Thames Valley NHS Improvement Programme, Article 3).

For most nurses, the simplest way of ensuring that any changes in medication happen correctly and without delay is to become adept at collaborating with professionals who work in the community such as GPs, pharmacists and community nurses. This will certainly help to prevent some of the problems that can occur after discharge. It could also reduce the number of drug-related re-admissions.

Fully independent nurse prescribers could, however, prescribe take-home medication as part of their discharge role. They could also contact their colleagues in the community with the exact details at the point of discharge. Non-prescribers could liaise with independent pharmacist prescribers in either secondary or primary care to fulfil this function. This would ensure continuation of the correct medication, even if hospital policies do not allow for more than a few days' supply of drugs on discharge.

Political initiatives on medication and discharge planning

Political initiatives

Three key policy areas have been selected for discussion here, with particular emphasis on how government policies positively or negatively impact upon the nurse's role and the effectiveness of patient discharge from hospital. Discharge planning continues to evolve rapidly and, in doing so, changes the interface with the pharmacist's role in both secondary and primary care settings.

Agenda for Change

Agenda for Change

Many healthcare professionals and other people working in secondary care settings have had their working practices affected by the implementation of the 'Agenda for Change' policy.

First, this policy has effectively reduced pharmacist hours by 5 per cent, thus cutting hospital pharmacy opening hours. Not all Trusts have developed strategies to circumvent this problem. And in some hospitals, attempts to stay within budget have resulted in additional reductions in pharmacy posts. This may well affect the time available for patients to engage in one-to-one discussion with a pharmacist about their medication on admission and discharge.

More positively, there is an increasing use of trained pharmacy technicians to oversee the practical aspects of ward drug supply. This extends to checking take-home medication, a role currently performed in many hospitals solely by the nurse discharging the patient. Using pharmacy technicians could free up nursing time, while still supporting other aspects of discharge from hospital.

Non-medical prescribing

Non-medical prescribing

Since the 1990s, nurses have been able to prescribe from a limited formulary as district nurses and health visitors. This has facilitated the supply of practical post-discharge necessities such as dressings, simple analgesia and laxatives. Extended independent and supplementary nurse prescribers have been in existence since 2002/3. Nurses are now able to prescribe from an increasingly extensive independent formulary for both minor ailments and more serious conditions, including some palliative care drugs, thus increasing post-discharge prescribing scope but also increasing the need for effective admission and discharge communication.

Supplementary prescribers, nurses and pharmacists and also,

potentially, radiographers, physiotherapists and podiatrists, can prescribe for any condition within their competence, under strict criteria agreed between themselves and an independent prescriber (usually a doctor). Again, this has many benefits but requires full communication between all prescribers on admission and discharge.

Independent prescribing for suitably trained nurses and pharmacists was announced in April 2006. This policy allows qualified individuals to prescribe from the whole of the British National Formulary (BNF). This should remove the need for debate about the legality of transcribing (copying) a patient's medication onto hospital medication sheets on admission, as such individuals could prescribe them legally. They could also prescribe any take-home medication required if systems for using PODs are not in operation.

Should suitably qualified staff members not be available to prescribe, Patient Group Directions (PGDs) could be set up to facilitate the continued supply of essential medication. This may also allow the supply of medication that would usually be unavailable in the community, e.g. IV solutions.

Information technology (IT)

The introduction of nationwide NHS IT systems has been long awaited. When implemented, these IT systems will allow real-time access to patient records for accredited personnel. This will mean that a patient's prescribed medication record can be transmitted directly from their GP practice to the hospital ward on admission, and the reverse process can occur on discharge. Community pharmacies will ideally be included in the information loop to ensure continuation of correct medication schedules after discharge.

All these measures should mean that fewer medication errors occur. However, this will still depend on the right information going to the right people and also, to a large extent, on the patient. History taking on admission will be able to focus more on the patient's knowledge and understanding of their medication, and any discrepancies will be noted and dealt with. Transmission of the patient's dispensed medication from their local pharmacy will also be possible. And, if patient registration with a specific pharmacy becomes the norm, hospital staff should get a better picture of how the patient is using, or not using, the medication their doctor has authorised on admission.

Post-discharge medication

**Post-
discharge
medication**

There is little point in changing medication, or any other aspect of therapy, in hospital if the changes are not maintained when the patient returns home. Community pharmacists, under the terms of their contracts, now undertake Medication Use Reviews (MURs) with their patients. Although any patient can request a review, as can healthcare professionals with the consent of the patient, they are especially useful for those individuals whose medication has changed or has become increasingly complex, or those who are at risk of confusion for other reasons. Reports are made to the patient's GP and these should help discharge nurses ensure that dosage changes are monitored, and any problems with changes in medication are identified.

Other ways of supporting patients at home might include telephone calls from the discharge nurse. These would provide opportunities to ask questions, give reminders of dosage schedules and pick up on any problems encountered.

Conclusion

In summary, nurses need to:
- Make sure they and the patient and/or their carers know what medication they were taking on admission
- Liaise with pharmacy as soon as possible so that discharge medication arrives on the ward without delay
- Ensure that ward patient records are clear in case other nurses have to deal with queries post discharge
- Explain the changes that have happened during the patient's stay
- Provide information about why and how to use the medication given on discharge
- Contact the patient's GP and community pharmacist to explain any medication changes made and to advise on the length of supply given on discharge

Clinical practice considerations

References

Ashford St Peters Hospital Policy for Nurse Checking and Issuing of Discharge Medication. (www.ashfordstpeters.nhs.uk/intranet/Ashford---/Publicatio/Policies-a/Procedure-for-nurse-checking-and-iss.doc)

Department of Health. (www.dh.gov.uk/PolicyAndGuidance/MedicinesPharmacyAndIndustry/Prescriptions/NonmedicalPrescribing/fs/en)

Thames Valley NHS Improvement Programme. 'Improving discharge – Medicines to take home' (Article 3). (www.tvip.nhs.uk/sharing-great-ideas)

Royal Pharmaceutical Society Briefing on Hospital Pharmacy, Summer 2006. (www.rpsgb.org.uk/pdfs/hosppharm21cbrief.pdf)

Section 3

Case studies

Chapter 10

Protocol or bespoke discharge plans?

Lynn Beun

In response to the publication of 'Ten key roles for nurses' (DoH 2000), a method of implementing nurse-facilitated discharge was developed at Brighton and Sussex University Hospitals NHS Trust (BSUH). A local Strategy for Nursing focus group, entitled 'Working in New Ways', led by the Assistant Director of Nursing, was established (BSUH NHS Trust 2002). This group examined a number of issues related to the scope of nursing practice. In BSUH NHS Trust, nurse-facilitated discharge was initially viewed as an expansion of the nurse's role.

A project plan was developed, identifying three main phases in the implementation of nurse-facilitated discharge for each ward:
1. Planning and preparation
2. Implementation on the ward
3. Review and evaluation

Phase 1: Planning and preparation

Planning and preparation

Before the implementation of nurse-facilitated discharge, the facilitator visited wards to help staff develop their local action plans. A simple document was used, entitled 'Nurse-facilitated discharge – is your ward ready?'. This document took the reader through a series of required actions, such as identifying the names of the ward consultants who supported nurse-facilitated discharge, and nominating competent nurses to undertake training and carry out the role. During this preparation phase, the ward teams also developed their own ward nurse-facilitated discharge checklist, which they later used when discharging the patient. This checklist

185

acted as a prompt but did not replace the need for critical thinking and problem solving.

Some Trusts use a universal discharge checklist on all wards. However, most staff prefer to design their own individual ward discharge lists because they are more specific to their own clinical practice. This process also gives staff the opportunity to engage with nurse-facilitated discharge before they have received their training.

The training was developed in collaboration with a nurse consultant from Birmingham Heartlands Hospital. Workshops were held once a month, and the teaching involved:

- Looking at the Trust organisational culture, the degree to which it is nurse-led or doctor-led, and how that has influenced the implementation within the Trust
- Examining clinical case studies to develop problem-solving skills (examples are included in this chapter)
- Exploring the legal and accountability issues raised by extended roles
- Self-evaluation of discharge skills, competency and reflection upon development needs

The preparation phase also included the establishment of a database of nominated nurses and a database to maintain patient details for audit purposes. This was required for the Clinical Negligence Scheme for Trusts (CNST) records. These databases provided evidence of training, which protected the Trust in cases where allegations to the contrary might be made. More importantly, ensuring that nurses are trained protects patients when nurses move ward or establishment.

Phase 2: Implementation

Implementing discharge

Thinking about carrying out nurse-facilitated discharge in the classroom or when reading a textbook is quite different from solving the problems of the patient in front of you. Different clinical situations may call for different approaches. At BSUH NHS Trust, the specialised needs of different patient groups mean that nurse-facilitated discharge needs to be implemented in different ways. The case studies below describe some of these approaches, and look at what worked well and what did not work so well.

Protocol or bespoke discharge plans?

Author's note: The following case studies are based on patients who were cared for at BSUH NHS Trust. In order to protect the identities of individual patients and maintain confidentiality, the case studies are synthesised from a large number of patients seen in clinical practice. They are not intended to bear any resemblance to actual individual patients.

Case study 1

Case study 1

Nurse-facilitated discharge and telephone follow-up for a patient having cataract surgery

Mrs A. was admitted to hospital for removal of a cataract and insertion of intra-ocular lens to the right eye under local anaesthetic. Two weeks before the planned operation date, Mrs A. was seen in the pre-operative assessment clinic. A health assessment was carried out to identify any potential problems in advance. The discharge plan was developed in the pre-operative assessment clinic as part of a patient care pathway, and discharge plans and transport arrangements were discussed. This enabled the patient and her family to make appropriate arrangements prior to her admission.

The care pathway continued when Mrs A. was admitted at midday and prepared for the operation that afternoon. Surgery went as planned and the surgeon stated in the notes that the nurse could discharge the patient and perform follow-up by telephone the next day. The staff nurse on duty delivered the care as planned in the care pathway, including a final checklist prior to discharge. The nurse informed Mrs A. that she would call her the next morning to carry out a phone check-up.

Later that afternoon Mrs A. was collected and taken home by a member of her family. The following day the staff nurse contacted the patient to review her progress. This was achieved by going through a list of questions documented on the care pathway to review clarity and brightness of vision, pain or discomfort, and check whether any nausea or vomiting had occurred. Mrs A. reported that she had felt some slight discomfort, but had not felt she needed to take any pain relief. This was recorded on the care pathway, and the nurse noted that this was within a normal limit on the pain scale. Mrs A. reported that her vision was brighter and clearer. The care pathway continued two weeks later at a post-operative clinic appointment.

Reflections

Before the implementation of nurse-facilitated discharge and telephone follow-up, medical staff saw the patients on the ward to perform a first day post-operative check. This was inconvenient for patients, as it meant that they had to return to hospital for a short visit. In addition, the post-operative check was carried out early in the morning, before medical staff went to attend clinics and theatre commitments. Having to return so early in the day was quite onerous for patients, some of whom had mobility difficulties.

The telephone check reduced the need for hospital transport, and thus enabled more patients to have their operations carried out as day case surgery. The implementation of nurse-facilitated discharge was enhanced by additional collaborative work with the pharmacy team and training for nurses on the provision of medication. Eye drops, which the patient needed to take home following surgery, were provided by the discharging nurse in a timely way.

Case study 2

Case study 2
Nurse-facilitated discharge for a patient with a chest infection

Mr B. was admitted to a medical ward with a chest infection. The estimated discharge date was three to four days from admission. Intravenous antibiotics were started. Mr B. took medication for hypertension, but his general health was otherwise good. On the post-take ward round he was seen by the consultant chest physician, who felt that Mr B. might be a suitable patient for nurse-facilitated discharge.

Discussing the patient's care needs with the multidisciplinary team, the consultant established parameters for discharge as follows:

- Patient apyrexial (temperature within normal limits) for 24 hours
- White cell count $< 15 \times 10^9$
- Established on oral antibiotics
- Patient has been seen by the Integrated Discharge Team (a multidisciplinary team, which includes physiotherapy,

occupational therapy and social work) and social care needs assessed

The staff nurse, who was trained to carry out nurse-facilitated discharge, coordinated the plan for the patient with the other members of the multidisciplinary team. As the patient recovered, the staff nurse was able to check that all the requirements had been met, and discharged the patient at the weekend. Previously, the patient might have had to stay in hospital until the consultant ward round on the Monday morning, to await a clinical decision.

Reflections

In the early stages of implementation, both medical and nursing staff found it difficult to write a discharge plan with clear parameters. One positive point was that the multidisciplinary team were involved in the development of the discharge plan. The blood count was specific, as was the need for the patient to be apyrexial for 24 hours. The discharge plan for a patient with a chest infection could have been improved by the addition of respiratory function criteria. For example, respiratory rate could have been an indicator that the patient was ready for discharge, as well as oxygen saturation levels or peak flow readings.

Case study 3

Case study 3
Nurse-facilitated discharge following percutaneous transluminal coronary angioplasty (PTCA)

Mrs C. suffered from ischaemic heart disease. She had an angiogram performed, which showed that she had an occluded right coronary artery. Following this procedure, a letter was sent to the patient informing her of her admission date. The letter also told her that nurse-facilitated discharge was being implemented, and explained what it was and what to expect. Mrs. C. was admitted to hospital for a percutaneous transluminal coronary angioplasty (PTCA) and stent to the right coronary artery later that day.

The procedure was carried out successfully, and Mrs C. returned to the ward and was monitored by nursing staff through the night. The consultant in charge documented in the care pathway notes that the patient was suitable for nurse-facilitated discharge. At 7 a.m. the nurse looking after

Mrs C. took an electrocardiogram (ECG) which showed normal sinus rhythm. The groin wound was checked and satisfactory. Observations of blood pressure, pulse and temperature were all within normal limits.

The nurse (who had undertaken training in nurse-facilitated discharge and was nominated by the ward manager to undertake the role) went through the discharge checklist. All criteria on the checklist were met. Mrs C. contacted her family and they were able to pick her up to take her home at 8 a.m. At 9 a.m. the nursing staff admitted the next patient to that bed.

Reflections

The preparation and leadership shown by the ward manager were valuable features of implementation on the ward. She took responsibility for developing a letter for patients that explained what nurse-facilitated discharge was and what to expect. She also identified the competencies she required from her staff and worked with the consultant to include nurse-facilitated discharge as part of the care pathway.

Case study 4

Case study 4
Nurse-facilitated discharge for a patient with complex health needs

One of the questions nurses frequently ask is 'Which patients are suitable for nurse-facilitated discharge?' Patients with multiple health and social problems, especially elderly medical patients, are sometimes thought to be unsuitable because they have complex care requirements. In fact the experienced nurse has an essential role to play in coordinating the discharge plan, liaising with other members of the multidisciplinary team and evaluating results. The value of nurse-facilitated discharge for such a patient is illustrated in the following case study.

Mr D. was a patient who lived in a nursing home. His medical history showed that he had multiple health problems, including Parkinson's disease, insulin-dependent diabetes mellitus and hypertension.

Mr D. was admitted to hospital following a two-day history of shortness of breath, pyrexia and increasing difficulties with swallowing. Mr D. was subsequently diagnosed as having a chest infection and had not been able to take the medication he required to control the symptoms of Parkinson's disease. This had led to swallowing difficulties, dehydration and confusion. Investigation and treatment were required, however, before the final diagnosis could be made and the discharge plan put together.

Following admission, the senior nurse worked with the other members of the multidisciplinary team to coordinate the investigations required and ensure that referrals were made to other disciplines. This included a review by the speech and language therapist and the physiotherapist.

When the diagnosis was confirmed and the treatment plan for the patient had been developed, the consultant identified that the patient was an appropriate subject for nurse-facilitated discharge. The team produced the following final discharge plan for the patient.

The nurse may discharge the patient when:

- The medical staff identify that the patient is medically fit for transfer and the medication to take away has been prescribed
- Physiotherapy assessment has been completed and the patient is able to walk up five steps
- The patient has been reviewed by the speech and language therapist prior to discharge
- The patient is able to tolerate thickened fluids (as defined by the Speech and Language therapist) and soft diet
- The patient's condition has been discussed with the nursing home and a discharge date has been agreed
- Transfer arrangements have been discussed with the next of kin

The multidisciplinary documentation included the use of an elderly care risk assessment checklist, which was completed within 24 hours of admission (BSUH NHS Trust 2004). The senior nurse liaised with the nursing home staff to explore their requirements and the possibility of transfer.

Reflections

The use of the discharge risk assessment checklist was valuable, because it supported the development of a care plan. The aspect that worked well for this patient was that the whole multidisciplinary team was involved in the development of the care plan to manage symptoms and identify the diagnosis. The final discharge plan was not completed until the diagnosis was known. In fact, although this was not recorded on the discharge plan, the patient was also referred to the nurse specialist for the elderly, who has a liaison role with nursing homes in the area. The plan could have been enhanced by adding the need for this referral. Further information about the discharge risk assessment checklist may be obtained from the author (see contact details at the end of this chapter).

Critical success factors: Ten golden rules

Critical success

During the early implementation stage, all ward staff were learning about nurse-facilitated discharge. From the lessons learnt, the following 'golden rules' were developed:

1. Obtain support from your senior management team. If the clinical management team support the development of nurse-facilitated discharge, implementation will be made easier.
2. Be flexible about your approach to nurse-facilitated discharge. For example, as the above case studies show, the method of nurse-facilitated discharge for patients having eye surgery is different from the approach taken with complex elderly patients.
3. Preparation and education are essential. Establish a practical training programme that meets your local needs. During the preparation stage, the team should also identify audit and evaluation methods.
4. Have a consultant 'champion'. Backing from medical staff and the enthusiasm of a consultant (who will support nurse-facilitated discharge at organisational level) are very important.
5. Be clear about which groups of patients may be included in nurse-facilitated discharge, and which groups may not be included.
6. Be explicit about which members of staff are competent to carry out nurse-facilitated discharge.
7. Do not develop a plan for nurse-facilitated discharge until you know what the diagnosis is for that patient. This does not mean that you cannot start the discharge planning process from admission. All nurses can start planning and making referrals, ensuring that investigations are carried out in a timely manner.

Protocol or bespoke discharge plans?

The multidisciplinary team should then develop the final discharge plan when a clear diagnosis is known. In the early stages of implementation on medical wards, the staff tried to develop discharge plans the day after admission.

8. Criteria for the discharge plan need to be very specific so that there is no scope for misinterpretation or misunderstanding in the decision-making process.

9. Nurse-facilitated discharge does not replace the multidisciplinary team – it complements it. The criteria for the discharge plan should include input from members of the multidisciplinary team. The ward multidisciplinary team meetings are the ideal setting for these discussions.

10. Persevere – progress will be made. During the early stages of implementation, progress seemed painfully slow, with only a small number of nurses actively undertaking the role. Gradually this changed, as more consultants, managers and senior nurses came to see the value of nurse-facilitated discharge, and as increasing numbers attended the training. The author would advise teams in the early implementation stage not to become discouraged, but to persist and learn from each patient. A huge amount of knowledge can be gained by examining a small number of patient case studies in detail.

Phase 3: Review and evaluation

Review and evaluation

During the early phase of implementation on each ward, the facilitator visited staff in order to support them, and to ensure that the correct procedures were being followed. When nurses discharged the patients they sent an audit form to the project facilitator, who would then check the patient's notes and outcomes.

Evaluation was carried out by examination of:

- The discharge plan and parameters described
- The nurse's discharge checklist
- Clinical outcomes for each patient
- Re-admission within two weeks
- Review of ward performance indicators (numbers of patients discharged before 11 a.m., days of the week patients discharged, and length of stay)

Case studies

Early audit results indicate the benefits of nurse-facilitated discharge in improving hospital flow and bed utilisation as follows:

- 61 per cent of nurse-facilitated discharge patients were discharged before 10a.m.
- 48 per cent of nurse-facilitated discharge patients were discharged at the weekend

To obtain staff views, a questionnaire was sent to all staff who were kept on the Trust database. This included staff who had attended the training but who had chosen not to undertake the discharge role, so that their views were taken into account and barriers to implementation were identified.

Case studies were drawn up to develop reflective learning skills and to use as problem-solving exercises for the training workshop.

During the review phase, changes were made to the ward discharge checklists, medical documentation and ward discharge processes as required, so staff could develop their practice further.

Conclusion

The implementation of nurse-facilitated discharge has been beneficial to Brighton and Sussex University Hospitals NHS Trust in a number of ways. The case studies show that care is now more focused on the needs of the patients, rather than around the timetables of hospital staff. For example, the patient with a chest infection could be discharged from hospital in a timely way. There was no need to wait for a decision because a clear plan was in place. The development of a clear discharge plan is useful for all members of the multidisciplinary team, including junior medical staff, as it makes the goals for the patient explicit.

The use of the discharge checklist acts as a prompt but does not replace the need for skilled clinical assessment of the patient and continuous evaluation.

During the initial development of nurse-facilitated discharge in Brighton and Sussex University Hospitals NHS Trust, it was viewed as a nursing role extension. As time passes, however, that perception is slowly changing and nurse-facilitated discharge is currently being written into nursing staff job descriptions as part of their nursing role. In the author's view, nurse-facilitated discharge of the patient will eventually become an integrated part of the nursing role.

References

Brighton & Sussex University Hospitals NHS Trust (2002). 'Strategy for Nursing'. Unpublished document, for local use.

Brighton & Sussex University Hospitals NHS Trust (2004). 'Elderly Care Proforma'. Unpublished care document, for local use.

Department of Health (2000). 'The NHS Plan: a plan for improvement, a plan for reform'. London: The Stationery Office.

If readers would like any further information about the Brighton & Sussex University Hospitals Trust documents they may contact the author of this chapter at the following address:
Service Improvement Team
Southpoint
8 Paston Place
Brighton BN2 1HA

Chapter 11

Nurse-facilitated discharge from Clinical Decisions Units (CDUs)

Bob McMaster

The recent emergence of specialist short-stay units has provided good opportunities for nurses developing discharge strategies. These units include Medical Assessment Units, Rapid Diagnosis and Treatment Centres, and Clinical Decisions Units (CDUs). Such units aim to have clearly structured management plans for patients. These plans have well-defined, criteria-based end points, which encourage early decisions regarding admission and discharge.

In Leeds, CDUs have been developed as an adjunct to the two emergency departments. These CDUs are used for patients with a range of conditions, to be managed on one of 19 evidence-based protocols (see below). The maximum planned length of patient stay is 24 hours. This allows for a short period of treatment and observation and rapid access to diagnostic investigations. Each condition has a timed review point at which a decision can be made about the patient's well-being and their physical, mental and social readiness for discharge. Decision-making is supported by flowcharts and pathways are incorporated into the protocols. These measures increase the consistency of patient management and reduce the risk of unsafe discharge.

CDUs provide two opportunities for nurse-facilitated discharge. One is through the use of protocols with defined criteria for discharge that can be utilised by medical staff or nurses. The other is through the development of nurse-led services, with nurses having inherent authority, accountability and responsibility for patient discharge. For the purposes of this chapter, the use, development and indications for discharge against protocols will be specifically explored.

Case studies

Using
protocols

> **Conditions managed on CDU by protocols**
>
> Asthma
> Anaphylaxis
> Cellulitis
> Community-acquired pneumonia
> Deliberate self-harm
> Deep vein thrombosis
> Headache
> Mild abdominal pain
> Minor gastro-intestinal bleed
>
> Minor head injury
> Non-traumatic chest pain
> Opioid toxicity
> Rapid response team assessment
> Renal colic
> Smoke inhalation
> Suspected pulmonary embolism
> Transient ischaemic attack
>
> Protocols available from EmiBank Medical Education Resource (2006).

Using protocols

Protocols, pathways, guidelines, flowcharts and management plans are terms that are sometimes used interchangeably to describe strategies for patient care. Protocols are used specifically for situations in which there are agreed structures, processes and outcomes for a precisely defined problem. Indeed, the Greek word protokollon means 'a note of agreement'. Within healthcare, a usable definition is offered by Field and Lohr (1992) as systematically developed statements to assist practitioner and patient decisions about appropriate healthcare for specific circumstances.

The development and use of protocols for patient management has been the subject of some criticism and debate. It is acknowledged that not all patients have straightforward conditions that lend themselves to the limitations of one pathway or protocol. Detractors argue that protocols can never provide answers for all eventualities and for all the decisions that practitioners have to make in what Schon (1991) describes as 'the swampy lowlands of practice'.

This is true, and it reinforces the point that protocols cannot and should not replace good clinical judgement in patient care. What protocols can offer is a safe and consistent standard of management for patients who meet defined inclusion criteria related to a given condition. Patients who do not meet the inclusion criteria, or who have more complex conditions and needs, are probably not suited to an environment such as a CDU.

Protocols can also help ensure that practice has a strong evidence base. In cases where strong evidence for a condition or treatment is lacking, protocols make it more likely that currently accepted best practice will be utilised. For example, there is an extremely limited evidence base for frequency of observations for patients with headache. However, the onset of new symptoms in acute onset headache is similar to that of head injury. National Institute for Clinical Excellence (NICE 2003) guidance on frequency of observations in head injury can therefore be applied as current suggested best practice.

For protocols to be acceptable to practitioners and patients, they should have the key attributes of good clinical guidance outlined by Rycroft-Malone (2002, Chapter 9). These are:

- Validity
- Cost-effectiveness
- Reproducibility
- Reliability
- Representativeness
- Clinical applicability
- Clinical flexibility
- Clarity
- Meticulousness
- Scheduled review
- Utilisation review

In Leeds, there is a consensus approach to the process of protocol development. A group is recruited that comprises members from the professional groups involved with implementing the protocols. These primarily include representatives from emergency department doctors and nurses, pharmacy, radiology, laboratories, and relevant medical specialties. Additional representatives are co-opted as required.

The group is given the task of reviewing current evidence and best practice related to diagnostic interventions, risk stratification, and treatment and observation strategies for each condition or patient group. Each protocol must demonstrate cost-effectiveness of management, and meticulous application of evidence and best practice. Where rapid or accelerated access to radiology or laboratory services are key to protocol delivery and patient management, an operational agreement is reached to guarantee timely access to the relevant services.

Recommendations are made to the group and a draft protocol is submitted for review. The protocol will include identification of relevant patients through inclusion and exclusion criteria, a structured management plan with suggested timescales for investigation and review, a flowchart for risk stratification, and criteria for admission or discharge. The draft protocol is piloted in practice for a short period to test validity, reliability, clarity and clinical applicability and flexibility, and any issues or problems are resolved. The final protocol is agreed and printed and disseminated into practice. There are planned reviews of all protocols once a year, or sooner if new evidence emerges.

Criteria for discharge are produced that are specific to each condition. These criteria take account of physiological improvement, mental well-being and social circumstances that permit discharge. For example, patients with asthma are recruited to a CDU and managed on an asthma protocol if they meet inclusion criteria of peak expiratory flow rate (PEFR) greater than or equal to 50 to 75 per cent of predicted best and signs of shortness of breath or wheeze. Treatment on the CDU includes, as required, bronchodilator inhalers/nebulisers and commencing steroids, and hourly observations of pulse, respirations, oxygen saturation and PEFR.

The factors underlying the current asthma attack are also explored. Patient review is at six hours and criteria for discharge are tested, of the patient being symptomatically improved with PEFR greater than 75 per cent and stable for two hours. Inhaler technique is checked and an adequate supply of inhaled B2 agonist and oral steroids is ensured. Contacts for emotional and psychological support are given if necessary, and the provision of safe and suitable social circumstances is discussed with the patient. The importance of compliance with treatment is emphasised and the patient is provided with clear written and verbal advice to return if their condition worsens. A GP letter is sent with the patient and posted to promote continuity of care.

The decision to discharge, and subsequent arrangements, can be made by either medical or nursing staff. Where there is diagnostic complexity or uncertainty, such as an ambiguous or deteriorating patient picture, then a medical review is sought. Providing medication to take home or discharge prescriptions can be facilitated through appropriate patient group directions and through the development of independent nurse prescribers. Further examples of discharge criteria can be found on the EmiBank website (EmiBank Medical Education Resource 2006).

Nurse-led services

Nurse-led services

When CDUs were being planned in Leeds there was a belief that they could be provided as a wholly nurse-led service. It soon became apparent that this would not be the case. The diagnostic complexity of some of the patient conditions required consistent input from medical staff, and were beyond the management experience of most CDU nurses at the time. The service was thus developed as a multidisciplinary unit. Subsequently, nurses have taken the lead in managing patients with a variety of conditions from arrival to discharge. These conditions have included suspected deep vein thrombosis (DVT), cellulitis, and deliberate self-harm. The remainder of this section will examine the impact of the nurse-led DVT service.

Around 800 patients per year present to the emergency departments in Leeds with suspected DVT. Before the establishment of CDUs, the patients were managed in an assortment of ways, with some being admitted to medical wards for investigation, while some were anti-coagulated and allowed home to await investigation. The opening of the CDUs and the launch of the DVT protocol meant that all these patients could be brought to a single location and that their management could be standardised. The centralisation of the service and the high caseload, as well as the presence of a CDU-dedicated nursing team, provided an ideal opportunity to develop DVT as a nurse-led service.

The first steps were to prepare a proposal for the Trust managers and nursing leads, to gather and ensure support for the expansion of scope of practice and the associated vicarious liability. Then an approach was made to local higher education institutions (HEIs) for suitable post-registration programmes and modules that would prepare the nurses for practice. Though the HEIs offered a range of specialist and advanced practice modules, none of them would have delivered the very specific preparation required to manage this group of patients. Therefore an education programme was developed in-house that focused on new skill and knowledge acquisition in key areas (see below).

Main components of in-house education for DVT management

- Professional, legal and ethical issues
- Related anatomy, physiology and pathophysiology
- Prevalence, origins and outcomes
- Differential diagnosis
- Pharmacology
- Systems for history-taking and clinical examination, documentation and communication
- Risk assessment and planned management using Wells

score and D-dimer/Ultrasound scanning (Wells *et al.* 1997)
- Ordering and interpreting investigations
- Treatment options, including medication via Patient Group Directions (PGD)
- Dispersal options – admission, home care, discharge
- Health promotion and advice

At the same time competencies were prepared, based on the agreed standards of practice stated in the protocol. There were also additional competencies related to the new skills of history-taking and clinical examination, and making safe decisions regarding patient dispersal to admission or discharge. Existing standards and competencies were drawn on for validity and reliability – in particular the Faculty of Emergency Nursing (2003) 'Competencies for Practice', and the Skills for Health Unit (2005) 'Competencies for Emergency Care'.

Supervision in practice was provided by the nurse consultant and middle-grade medical staff. This consisted of direct supervision of the first two or three cases undertaken by each CDU nurse, then indirect supervision for a further seven to ten cases. In order to guarantee safety, all patients had their case notes and management reviewed prior to discharge. After a minimum of ten cases the nurses submitted their protocol notes for audit against the competency statements.

When the required standard of management was demonstrated consistently the nurses made a self-declaration of competence. This indicated that they felt ready to accept responsibility and accountability for the management, from admission to discharge, of patients with suspected DVT. Further supervision and guidance was available as required for the nurses. This support helped them to progress from being not merely competent but also confident in their patient management. This further advance (from competence to confidence) took from three to six months, depending on individual learning styles and the availability of DVT patients.

The benefits of the service can be demonstrated in several ways. For the emergency service, 88 per cent of 1,068 patients attending in one year with suspected DVT were managed through the nurse-led scheme. A total of 12 per cent could not attend the CDU either because it was full or because there wasn't a suitably experienced nurse available to make the patient assessment.

Of those attending the scheme:

- 83 patients were admitted because of large DVTs or complications
- 42 were referred to the nurse-led anti-coagulation outreach service for management at home
- 516 were discharged to their GP
- 283 were discharged and brought back to a planned clinic appointment
- 16 took their own discharge against advice

The overall discharge rate from the nurse-led DVT service was 89 per cent.

All patients attending the nurse-led service have been offered the alternative option of seeing a doctor. To date, only one patient has taken this option. In a satisfaction survey, 96 per cent of patients reported that the CDU service was good, very good or excellent. Reports of dissatisfaction concerned lengths of waiting times for investigations and the quality of hospital food.

An audited comparison of management by CDU nurses with management by emergency department medics revealed no difference in overall process time for patients. However, there was good use of Well's score by nurses, preventing one-third of patients from having unnecessary ultrasound scans. There was also good diagnosis and identification of differential problems, a better standard of documentation and increased consistency of management by nurses. CDU nurses report a high level of satisfaction in their DVT roles and their expertise is recognised within the emergency department, with nurses providing an opinion or review for other staff.

Overall, the nurse-led scheme has provided benefits for patients, for nurses and for the emergency service.

Conclusion

Nurse-facilitated discharge from CDUs can develop in two ways. One is by including clear discharge criteria within all the protocols that can be accessed by both medical and nursing staff. The second is through the development of nurse-led services, in which nurse-facilitated discharge is an integral part. The latter also offers additional benefits to the emergency service, to nurses working under the scheme, and to patients.

Case studies

References

EmiBank Medical Education Resource (2006). Leeds Teaching Hospitals NHS Trust. (www.leedsteachinghospitals.com/sites/emibank/clinicians/cdu/index.php)

Faculty of Emergency Nursing (2003). 'Competencies for Practice'. London: Royal College of Nursing.

Field, M.J. & Lohr, K.N. (eds) (1992). *Clinical Practice Guidelines: Directions for a New Program.* Washington: National Academy Press.

National Institute for Clinical Excellence (2003). 'Head injury: Triage, assessment, investigation and early management of head injury in infants, children and adults'. London: NICE.

Rycroft-Malone, J. (2002). 'Clinical Guidelines' in Thompson, C. & Dowding, D. (2002). *Clinical Decision Making and Judgement in Nursing.* Edinburgh: Churchill Livingstone.

Schon, D. (1991). *The Reflective Practitioner* (2nd edn). New York: Basic Books.

Skills for Health Unit (2005). 'Competencies for Emergency, Urgent and Unscheduled Care'. (Available at www.skillsforhealth.org.uk).

Wells, P.S., Anderson D.R., Bormanis, J. *et al.* (1997). 'Value of assessment of pre-test probability of deep vein thrombosis in clinical management'. *Lancet,* 350 (9094), 1795–1798.

Chapter 12

A project-managed approach to nurse-facilitated discharge within a Trauma and Orthopaedic Unit

Karen Tongue

In the light of increasing demands on acute hospital beds, and the recognised benefits to patients who are discharged in a timely way, this chapter looks at the way a project-managed approach within a Trauma and Orthopaedic (T&O) Unit brought about sustainable changes to practice. It illustrates how the Trauma wards have delivered benefits for the multidisciplinary team, as well as the desired benefits for patients and their carers. This chapter discusses:

- How to use a project-managed approach
- How multidisciplinary team-facilitated discharge differs from nurse-facilitated discharge
- Tips for success

Background

In August 2004 the Department of Health (DoH 2004a) published a best practice document, 'Achieving timely "simple" discharge from hospital: A toolkit for the multidisciplinary team'. This cited areas of good practice throughout the country, providing practical steps that could be adopted.

The Chief Nursing Officer named the ability to admit and discharge patients with specified conditions and within agreed protocols, underpinned by appropriate knowledge, as one of the 'ten key roles' that would effectively modernise nursing (DoH 2000).

Guidance was also issued by the Modernisation Agency to improve care of orthopaedic patients (DoH 2005). This document specifically stated that 'Supporting discharge schemes can work extremely well – a number of teams offering this service for their joint replacement patients have now extended the service to patients admitted with fractured neck of femur'. It was an encouraging document, which emphasised that discharge should be an integral part of any care pathway in order to achieve an impact on length of stay and fast-track 'those who would recover quickest'.

What does timely discharge mean for Trauma patients?

Timely discharge

In 2004, I was a senior sister working in a 50-bed Trauma unit and was offered the opportunity for a fresh challenge. At the same time, the T&O Directorate team were concerned that Trauma patients were staying in hospital for unnecessarily extended periods of time. This not only affected the Directorate's ability to manage admissions within the bed capacity, but also had a negative impact on patients. I was asked to explore what I thought could be done about this, and to formulate a project proposal to manage the change that was envisaged. This proposal would be presented to the Directorate for approval.

Within the Trust, other projects were underway and a Discharge Practice Group had been created to drive forward innovative new discharge practices across the Trust in a coordinated way. This enabled the T&O team to legitimately seek support for changing discharge practice from elsewhere in the Trust. The project envisaged by the T&O Directorate required measurable outcomes, both in terms of quality gains and financial benefits.

The project manager was supernumerary (not counted in with the staffing allocations), allowing the close monitoring of practice changes and the precise identification of which areas of practice needed to be addressed, particularly the obstacles to discharge as they existed prior to any changes (see below). The project manager needed to network with the members of the multidisciplinary team. This is important when considering change that will impact across a whole team.

Identified obstacles to timely discharge:
- Lack of consultant management plan
- Access to rehabilitation beds

- Timely availability of tablets to take home
- Perception that there was insufficient time to plan discharge
- Five-day working of occupational therapists
- Lack of joined-up professional team working

How does a project-managed approach work?

Over the years, a number of discharge initiatives have been introduced and then forgotten. Many have never developed beyond the planning stages, whilst others raised expectations of change but somehow failed at the final hurdle. When considering the project I was very mindful of this, recognising the need to engage the team in change that was sustainable. Equally, the proposed changes had to offer benefits to individual professional groups as well as meeting the needs of individual patients, the Directorate and the Trust as a whole.

The Department of Health toolkit 'Achieving timely "simple" discharge from hospital' (DoH 2004a) states that discharges from acute hospitals can be divided into 80 per cent simple discharges, with the remaining 20 per cent requiring more complex issues to be resolved. With this in mind, I reviewed our current patient group and found that 42 per cent of the patients required a complex discharge package.

I regarded 'complex' discharges as those patients who required a referral to Social Care (for social support or placement) and those patients who required rehabilitation from occupational therapists and physiotherapists. I believe that these 42 per cent of patients were representative of many Trauma patients in acute care. For example, many of them were elderly and frail with co-morbidities, and many were living alone.

The group of patients with fractured neck of femur often presented major challenges for the Trauma team. It was in this group that the Directorate wished to see a significant reduction in length of stay. It was also recognised that this group of patients had an increasing morbidity and mortality rate if their discharge was delayed. This was also demonstrated in the Dr Foster report (provided by an independent health service research organisation) and was a concern to everyone involved in the patient's care pathway.

Case studies

The proposed changes would enable the discharge of patients within the Trauma wards to become driven by a recognised process. This would remove the belief that discharge practice was often disjointed and dependent on too many individual variables. For example, the standard of discharge practice might previously have been influenced by whether or not experienced nurses were on duty, what day of the week it was (which would influence the volume of discharges), or when and which particular consultant teams were due to do their rounds.

What were the objectives of the project?

The project proposal was influenced by the following factors:

Objectives of project

- National agenda
- Local agenda
- Need to dispel some myths about discharge
- Need for a multidisciplinary approach
- Trust and Directorate support
- Recognition that this needed to be the catalyst for future developments

As the project was seen as a catalyst for long-term investment in multidisciplinary team working, clear objectives needed to be established. The three main project objectives were to:

1. Improve bed flow and bed capacity usage
2. Introduce nurse-facilitated discharge
3. Introduce a consultant post-take management plan

The success of the project very much depended on supporting teams in creating a way forward. It was felt that this could be best achieved by the project facilitator working within the multidisciplinary team but with supernumerary status. In order to fund this, I needed to be creative with my project proposal. I had to demonstrate that, by reducing length of stay for a group of Trauma conditions, a financial saving could be achieved. This evidence would then be used to support the project facilitator role.

I took the bold step of deciding that introducing nurse-facilitated discharge could reduce length of stay by one day, across four patient condition groups. Based on 2004-2005 data, I estimated that 126 bed days could be saved in the first six months of the project (see over).

Patient group	Number of patients	Current length of stay in days	Estimated new length of stay in days	Potential bed days saved
#ankles	56	8.25	7.25	56
#wrists	47	8.14	7.14	47
#metacarpals	16	2.34	1.34	16
#metatarsals	7	4.64	3.64	7
Totals	126			126

This potential saving of bed days would fund my 0.6wte Grade G project facilitator post. It was difficult to demonstrate proven savings as I was not proposing to close beds, reduce establishments, or operate on more elective cases (elective cases were managed on a different site). I realised that I was asking the Directorate to take a risk!

However, I was able to identify clear benefits for three groups, namely, patients and their carers, the Trust and the multidisciplinary team. These benefits are detailed below.

Benefits of nurse-facilitated discharge for orthopaedic patients
For patients and their carers:
- Clearly identified responsibilities prior to discharge
- Greater involvement in the decision-making process
- Realistic expectations
- Improved patient experience

For the Trust:
- Improved patient flow
- Improved communication between the Trust and other agencies
- Reduced complaints
- Improvements in Dr Foster data
- Competent skilled workforce
- Improved patient experience

For the multidisciplinary team:
- New role development in line with NHS Knowledge and Skills Framework
- Obtaining new skills
- Improved job satisfaction
- Autonomous practice
- 'Ten key roles' for nurses (as specified by the Chief Nursing Officer)

To realise this vision of the project and how it would achieve the desired benefits, a great deal of conviction was required on the part of the project facilitator. Three further vital factors were identified, namely: a good plan, a full project team (see below) and strong leadership skills to maintain staff commitment to the project. It is said that a good plan should 'comfort the disturbed and disturb the comforted'.

Agreeing the project plan

It was important to involve the teams at the beginning of the process. In order to achieve this, a project group with representation from each professional group was required. A project leader was also appointed to take overall responsibility for the delivery of the project outcomes.

An initial meeting went well with full representation, although this was not easy to achieve in a busy clinical environment. Minutes were taken and individual actions and timescales were agreed upon. Each objective was explored and the types of actions that would be required were also clearly identified. It was decided that further communication would take place through bi-monthly Directorate progress reports, ward meetings and newsletters.

There was a little scepticism within the team but mainly excitement that this was an opportunity to introduce real change by looking at the way professional groups worked with other professional groups. Each member of the group was charged with discussing the outcomes of each meeting with their colleagues, and bringing any feedback to the following meeting.

The project team
Project leader: Associate specialist surgeon
Project facilitator: Senior trauma sister
Senior occupational therapist
Senior physiotherapist
Clinical nurse specialist
Ward nurses
Outreach team members

The role of project facilitator

Having formulated the project proposal, the next stage was to verify the attainability, measurability and desired outcomes of the project. In addition, the plan needed to encompass all the

Facilitating

elements of successful change management, such as adequately identifying champions from the ward areas and assessing whether we would be able to rely upon their engagement throughout the project. As the facilitator, I explored the commitment that each individual would need to give to the group to achieve the outcomes required.

An open forum was created in which individuals were able to participate fully and feel that their opinions were valued. Membership of the forum was based on whether I felt an individual had demonstrated an ability to be a team player. They also needed to have shown an interest in inter-professional working and demonstrated a commitment to changing discharge in practice.

It became obvious within the first few weeks that there were high expectations within the ward teams and also within the Directorate and the organisation as a whole. This acted as an inspiration to progress the work.

Reviewing work already underway in other areas of the Trust was a crucial part of my role as facilitator. This process enabled me to access all relevant resources and bring them to the attention of the project forum. I was already a firm believer in not 're-inventing the wheel', and it became evident that progress against our objectives had already been made elsewhere. For example, a 'Nurse-led discharge protocol', a 'Discharge pathway for patients requiring rehabilitation', and 'Post-take management plans' had already been formulated (Lees, Allen & O'Brien 2006).

It was evident that a multi-professional 'joined-up' approach was needed. I was aware that each professional group worked within their professional guidelines, with a common belief that each was doing everything possible to achieve timely discharge. This project required a change in thinking by the whole team, whereby discharge would became an integral part of daily ward activity.

The three keys to success were:
- Engaging expertise
- Joined-up approaches within the hospital
- Accessing best practice

Case studies

Watching the changes unfold

Watching the changes

Having an opportunity to stand back and observe practice had given me a chance to see how we could create working patterns that would impact on timely discharge. One early change we made was to introduce a mini multidisciplinary team meeting at 8.30a.m. in each ward, where each patient's progress against their estimated discharge date could be discussed. This worked extremely well, although for those involved it was not always easy to find time for an additional 20-minute meeting amid the pressure of morning activities.

I also asked the ward teams to look at the structure of the weekly multidisciplinary team meeting, which traditionally lasted for about 45 minutes. I was aware that these meetings were time-consuming for everyone and did not always identify the actions required for individual patients to achieve their timely discharge. Changes to these meetings included recording outcomes in the daily round book to improve communication. This allowed easy identification of who was responsible for required actions. It was also agreed that an intermediate care facilitator would be invited to the meetings. This facilitator would then be able to take referrals directly from the meeting.

What did the project achieve and what are the associated issues?

Achievements and issues

The formal evaluation of the project is currently underway. However, some major changes in practice have already been identified.

1. Trauma Outreach Service

As a result of the project, the multidisciplinary team decided to explore the possibility of having a Trauma Outreach Service. By involving members of the Orthopaedic Outreach Service in our project group, a protocol was created and the new service was introduced as a six-month pilot. This additional outreach service has resulted in significant savings in bed days across the full range of Trauma conditions in the first four months. If this trend continues, it will become a permanent addition to the discharge options for Trauma patients within the Trust.

2. Nurse-facilitated discharge protocols

These protocols have been developed and are ready to implement. Many of the staff on the wards have received training in the legal and professional aspects involved. Gaining absolute competence is an issue, linked to personal development plans. And individual appraisals, linked to career progression, will be the next step. These developments are inextricably linked with the NHS 'Knowledge and Skills Framework' (DoH 2004b).

Discharge competencies have already been developed, and will form a vital framework for the implementation stage. Supporting staff through the development of competency in practice has already been a challenge, despite expert support within the Trust. Regardless of the support available, we need to be able to demonstrate objectivity in which individuals we support, and when and how we support them. At this point we have had to put this on hold, as a number of staff have progressed in their careers and left the ward. Clearly, when embarking on a project of this magnitude, it is of paramount importance to consider not only the initial training required but also the ongoing needs of the workforce.

3. Discharge pathways for fractured neck of femur patients

These were developed early in the project, in collaboration with the ward multidisciplinary team, alongside the elderly care consultant responsible for in-house patient rehabilitation. This change is now embedded in practice. It has proven to be a positive development, and the rehabilitation potential of individual patients is now regularly assessed by the multidisciplinary team and consultant. This allows changes to the discharge destination to be made, to the benefit of the patient.

4. Consultant post-take management plans

Such plans had previously been introduced within a Medical Directorate, with recognised benefits to the post-take ward rounds. By adapting this document to meet the needs of Trauma patients, this approach could be introduced to the Trauma consultants. They recognised the obvious benefits of documenting a clear plan of care for each patient on the post-take round, including discharge pathway, estimated length of stay and required surgery. Each set of notes had a bright yellow plan inserted prior to the round, requiring the team to complete the plan rather than the traditional entry written in the notes. Each consultant was introduced to the idea and feedback was positive.

However, the use of the plan depended on a nurse reminding and encouraging the medical team to complete the form. Old habits are hard to break; and medical rounds are often rushed, because of the pressure to arrive in theatre or clinic on time. Therefore, although it often appears easy to transfer an idea to another clinical area, getting the consultants to complete the plans proved the hardest part and adversely affected the success of their implementation in practice. This is an aspect of the project that needs revisiting. As the positive gains outweigh the difficulties, a different approach may be needed. For instance, it might be feasible for the clinical nurse specialist or discharge co-ordinator to complete the form and the surgeon to acknowledge its appropriate completion by signing it at a later point, thus not precluding the plan.

5. Theatre discharge plans

Throughout the development of the nurse-facilitated protocol it was clear that an accurate medical plan was needed. The project group felt that this could be achieved whilst the patient was in theatre, as the surgeon was best placed to make decisions on discharge date, follow-up, and whether a cast was required prior to discharge. This plan has been added to the operation notes, removing the need to complete an extra form. Discharge medication can also be prescribed in theatre. It is envisaged that this will be an addition to the surgeon's usual operating responsibilities, accepting that discharge planning is part of everyone's responsibilities.

The post-take plans and the theatre plans have not yet been accepted as part of everyday practice and still rely heavily on nursing expertise and enthusiasm to prompt the teams to deliver the best outcome. This is a challenge and, whilst acknowledging the heavy workload of our medical colleagues, this is an area that will be reviewed with a re-launch planned.

What are the positive outcomes of the project?

Positive outcomes

This has proved to be a multifaceted project in which ideas for good practice have continually evolved. The project has delivered progress beyond that originally anticipated against each of the three main objectives (see p. 208). Although it has yet to be formally evaluated, the project has resulted in a variable reduction in length of stay for some of our patients. I believe that there will be further reductions in length of stay when the 'Nurse-facilitated discharge protocol' is launched in the next few weeks. The re-launch of the discharge management plans will undoubtedly contribute to further improvements in care and possibly length of stay reduction.

Some of the key achievements are listed below. These are best regarded as qualitative outcomes. As such, they are not very easy to measure. Yet, without these aspects, the issues raised would probably not have been addressed and solutions might not have been identified. Each forms a step in its own right towards the overall objective of improved discharge practice and reducing length of stay.

Key achievements

- Inter-professional working
- Breaking down traditional barriers
- Working with new colleagues
- Pride in what has been achieved
- Enthusiasm for trying new ways of working
- Recognition of results within the wider organisation
- Work being adapted in other areas of the organisation
- Self-belief of ward teams
- Recognition of benefits of nurse-led initiatives
- Greater understanding of each other's roles
- A knowledge of how this project fits into the national NHS agenda

Conclusion

A lot of tenacity has been required during this project, as at times it felt as though we were not going to succeed. At these times, the forum needed to remain focused, supporting the ward teams when things were notoriously difficult and re-evaluating the steps that were needed to reach the goals. In an ever-changing environment, we recognised that the need to be flexible was of paramount importance. It was vital to realise that individuals' workloads could vary and the project objectives could not always take priority in a busy clinical setting.

When the project proposal was written it was not envisaged that we would have a Trauma Outreach Service. (Many had said before that it couldn't be done.) But, by using a project-managed approach, a significant sustainable change in practice occurred. More work still needs to be done if discharge planning is to become a transparent process. In this case, the project had to start at the point where practitioners were. The project facilitator's role was to support them through change, acting as the eyes and ears of staff, and being both the catalyst and the promulgator of future change.

References

Department of Health (2000). 'The NHS Plan: a plan for improvement, a plan for reform'. London: The Stationery Office.

Department of Health (2004a). 'Achieving timely "simple" discharge from hospital: A toolkit for the multidisciplinary team'. London: The Stationery Office. (www.dh.gov.uk)

Department of Health (2004b). 'The NHS Knowledge and Skills Framework'. London: The Stationery Office. (www.dh.gov.uk)

Department of Health (2005). 'Faster access for orthopaedic patients: Best practice guidance'. London: The Stationery Office.

Lees, L., Allen, G. & O'Brien, D. (2006). 'Using post-take ward rounds to facilitate simple discharge'. *Nursing Times*, 102 (18) 28–30. (www.nursingtimes.net)

Chapter 13

Nurse-facilitated weekend discharges

Andrea Field

Background

This case study is based on a project undertaken within a large NHS Acute Foundation Trust. For many years, the Trust had battled to find a solution to the effective management of bed capacity over the winter months. Although additional 'flexible' wards were opened over this period, Monday mornings were chaotic, as patients were housed in Endoscopy and the Day Surgery Unit due to the lack of bed capacity. This resulted in the cancellation of elective procedures. More importantly, it led to poor quality of care, as the most acutely ill patients were being cared for in environments that were not 'fit for purpose'.

When analysing the pattern of discharges it became clear that there were minimal discharges over the weekend. In addition, the day of the week with the highest discharge rate was Monday, which suggested that some of these patients could have been discharged over the weekend. Based on this information, the Matron for Acute Medicine was given the task of leading a project across medicine to encourage nurse-facilitated weekend discharges.

The project: Stage 1

The project began in December 2002 and the model chosen was a 'top down' approach to change management. This approach was chosen because it was the quickest to implement and did not involve changing individual cultures at ward level. The project leader identified four interested senior nurses (band 7), who agreed to work over the weekends across medicine and identify patients suitable for nurse-facilitated discharge and then facilitate the discharge process. In addition, the physician on call each Saturday agreed to provide medical advice to enable discharges to happen.

Initially, time was spent on defining what nurse-facilitated discharge actually meant. The debate continued until the project leader concluded that the definition was not the most crucial success factor for the project, and that the actual process of discharging a patient at the weekend should be the prime focus. With this in mind, the project began.

The senior nurses collated the number of patients who, through their intervention, had been discharged over the weekend. The weekend actually began on Friday afternoon, when the senior nurse would trawl the wards and identify patients who could potentially go home over the weekend. The senior nurse would liaise with the patient's medical team to finalise the discharge plans. Over the weekend, the senior nurse would then check that these patients had been discharged. The senior nurse would also liaise with the consultants on their post-take ward rounds on Saturday and Sunday mornings to identify further patients who only required a short period of in-patient treatment.

Project data

Project data

The overall figures were evaluated by the project leader each week and the figures were sent to the key stakeholders, namely the Chairman, the Deputy Director of Nursing and the Operational Director for Medicine. Between December 2002 and November 2003, 2,257 patients were discharged over the weekend via the project. However, the project was expensive to maintain, as we were paying the senior nurses to do additional shifts at prime weekend rates. In addition, the senior nurses lost momentum as they had undertaken the project in addition to their full-time roles and were paid via the Trust's nurse bank. The project to date had resulted in Endoscopy and the Day Procedures Unit not being used inappropriately throughout the period from December 2002 to November 2003. However, regardless of these benefits, the project was not sustainable at this point.

The project: Stage 2

**The project:
Stage 2**

Following a discussion with the key stakeholders, it was decided that a 'bottom up' approach should now be applied. Each ward was given responsibility for their own weekend discharges. In addition, they were given a target to achieve, agreed in advance with the matron for each area. Initially, this resulted in an increase in discharges, particularly on a Friday. This indicated that the nursing staff were focusing on discharge.

Data collection was not robust, as there were differences in the way nurse-facilitated discharge was interpreted and counted by individuals, and each ward reported its own achievement – with little external validation. Progress was not sustained and eventually, by November 2004, the numbers of weekend discharges had decreased. However, it is important to note that the numbers were not reduced to the levels seen before the project began. This indicated that there had been some sustainable change.

Nurse-facilitated discharge protocols

Protocols

While the weekend discharge project was underway, a separate project was being undertaken to develop disease-specific nurse-facilitated discharge protocols. This was a complex process centring on the admission and nurse-facilitated discharge of patients with asthma.

The asthma protocol, when finalised, proved to be ineffective. The criteria were too specific and the protocol did not work in conjunction with the patient's disease processes. The protocol indicated specific physical criteria that had to be in place before the patient's discharge. For example, the patient needed to have been transferred from nebulisers to inhalers and have maintained an oxygen saturation rate on air of above 90 per cent. However, many chronic asthma sufferers have several other co-morbidities. They may be stable with oxygen saturation rates of below 90 per cent and are often discharged with these lower levels. Therefore the protocol actually paralysed the discharge process and was soon discarded.

From this work, it was clear that nurse-facilitated discharge had to be based on parameters for individual patients set by their medical or specialist nurse teams.

Case studies

What were the limiting factors in the nurse-facilitated weekend discharge project?

The factors limiting the progress of the project were as follows:

- An assumption was made that nurses knew how to discharge patients. This was not the case.
- Fundamental systems of work did not change, and therefore the project had limited success and sustainability.
- Ambiguous entries in the medical records made it impossible to instigate nurse-facilitated discharge.
  For example, one entry stated 'discharge over the weekend if OK' and another said 'aim for home early next week'.
- There was no 'win win' for the nursing staff. If they could discharge their most independent patients over the weekend, acutely ill, dependent patients would replace them. Where was the incentive?
- Any project like this can be limited by the lack of seven-day working amongst allied health and social care professionals outside nursing. For example, a patient who needs a stair assessment on a Friday afternoon, prior to discharge, may well wait until Monday for this to happen.
- Throughout the project it became clear that some consultants were reluctant to make decisions about discharge if the patient was not under their care.
  The Trust needs to develop ways of engaging all consultants if length of stay is to be reduced and timely discharge achieved
- There was a lack of ownership of the change process. Initially a 'top down' approach was used and failed. Later a 'bottom up' approach was used, with no education or preparation, and it also failed.
- The organisation wanted an immediate answer to the problem of weekend discharges, which was not realistic. If time had been allowed to plan and implement a more robust system then the results could have been improved and more easily maintained. Change management approaches were, in a sense, thrown at the project, when what was needed was time and the opportunity to gradually change the way professionals worked.

What are the keys to success in implementing this type of project?

- Don't assume that nurses have the required knowledge; check first.
- Establish a model of change management that is robust and stick to it. The question to ask is: 'If the project leader left tomorrow, would the change be sustained?'
- Always consider providing an incentive when asking staff to work harder. Would the nurses be more willing to discharge patients if they had their own patients admitted, rather than outliers from other specialities?
- Establish clear discharge criteria before embarking on nurse-facilitated discharge. If the discharge requirements are unknown, how can nurse-facilitated discharge be implemented?
- Involve all disciplines in any project relating to patient care. One discipline alone cannot make a significant change.
- Challenge the provision of services from departments such as pharmacy and radiology, as they are key in instigating any significant change to the prompt discharge of patients.
- Look at core systems of working before instigating change to ensure that changes will result in effective and sustainable improvements.
- Always consider the patient. Never embark on a project for the sake of meeting targets rather than improving the quality of patient care.

What is the current focus on discharge?

The current focus is on strengthening the overall management plans for discharge from the point of admission (Lees *et al.* 2006). For example, patient management plans have been introduced for post-take ward rounds. These plans include the setting of an estimated date of discharge (EDD), the criteria for discharge, and the estimated length of stay

This system requires medical staff, in particular, to work differently. It will therefore take time for them to actively engage with this new type of documentation. The acute medical consultants have adapted to this method of working but other specialities are proving to be more difficult to convince. When EDD and criteria for discharge are used effectively then bed capacity can be planned more accurately, and discharge will occur seven days a week in a timely and effective manner.

References

Lees, L., Allen, G. & O'Brien, D. (2006). 'Using post-take ward rounds to facilitate simple discharge'. *Nursing Times*, 102 (18) 28–30. (www.nursingtimes.net)

Chapter 14

Simple discharge illustrated

Ann Edgar

This chapter will explore what is regarded as a simple discharge. It will also look at the key principles and activities that underpin discharge practice and offer suggestions to improve practice. It is written from the perspective of a modern matron within the elderly care directorate of an acute hospital setting.

The modern matron's role is very broad and is constantly evolving to encompass new aspects of risk, governance and clinical standards. Above all, the modern matron is responsible for the coordination of safe, high-quality care. Discharge planning is an integral part of this role, in order to promote safe, effective and timely discharge. Moreover, discharge planning remains a key indicator of hospital performance across a range of interrelated issues that impact upon discharge practice. Yet, despite the prominence of the matron's role, feedback from patients' relatives (through both informal and formal processes) indicates that Trusts do not always get it right. Matrons need to be both energetic and assiduous in showing leadership and improving the knowledge and skills of their nursing staff.

Whether a discharge is simple or complex, the principles behind the process of discharge remain the same. In addition, although the focus of different perspectives of discharge may be presented in a contemporary manner, the accelerated pace of change has influenced the profile of discharge practices.

Defining simple discharge

Simple discharge

Around 80 per cent of discharges from hospital are said to be 'simple' (DoH 2004). However, this figure can be very different in clinical areas involving patients with ongoing healthcare needs, or where patients may be heavily dependent on services that support discharge from hospital to home. For example, the elderly care rehabilitation ward in Birmingham Heartlands Hospital recently represented the converse picture, with 80 per cent complex discharges and 20 per cent simple. Hence the age of a patient and length of stay in hospital may not always determine whether or not a discharge is regarded as simple. The components determining the nature of discharge include: complexity of assessment, support needed, number of professionals involved and actions required.

Simple discharge	Complex discharge

• Often only a single disciplinary assessment is required
• Support of relatives can be assumed
• Existing care package may already be in place
Or:
• No ongoing care needs are identified
• Discharge planning needs are typically met by simple actions, e.g.:
  • Tablets to take out
  • Transport
  • Arranging appointments
  • Engaging district nursing services
• Estimated date of discharge may be relatively easy to predict, with few variables to manage
	• Multidisciplinary assessment required
	• Financial assessment required
	• May not have a family support network
	• Support was not required previously
	Or:
	• Increased level of support now required
	Or:
	• Change of residence now required
	And:
	• Continuing healthcare needs have been identified
	• Discharge liaison nurses are pivotal to the discharge planning
	• Multidisciplinary team meetings are central to the planning

A few considerations regarding simple discharges

The assessment process

In a recent documentation audit within the elderly care directorate the initial assessment of a patient contained inaccurate information. It had been noted that the patient lived in a residential home. On transfer to the ward, this information had been added to the nursing assessment. The residential home had thus become the expected discharge destination.

It was not until seven days later, when a member of the nursing team contacted the 'residential home', that they discovered it was actually sheltered housing. This lack of accurate assessment (at the outset) delayed discharge by another five days, to allow time for home visits and modifications to the environment. This example demonstrates poor communication and poor coordination throughout the process by the members of the team involved.

Communication within the ward

Communication

To ensure effective discharge communication, registered nurses require knowledge, skill, experience and the ability to appreciate different situations from the patient's perspective. Although communication skills can be taught, they also require practice. Reflection, and action on reflection, involves continually evaluating good and less good discharge practice and learning from experience. Senior nurses (certainly band 6 and above) have a vital part to play in guiding their teams, through such experience, to become proficient communicators.

New roles may also be helpful, especially where the turnover or complexity of patients is a dominant feature of the ward environment. For example, in elderly care a 'communication nurse role' has been developed and piloted within one ward area. This role is specifically aimed at senior registered nurses who coordinate all communications between the various team members on a daily basis. The role is still in its infancy and continues to evolve (see below). But it has already increased the emphasis placed on discharge practice and may bring about a reduction in patients' length of stay by ensuring that vital communications are not omitted and actions are progress-chased. This example demonstrates that strong clinical leadership at ward level is a vital factor in improving the discharge process

Before and after establishment of the communication nurse role

Before	After
• Fragmented communications	• Consistent approach to communications
• Limited opportunity for teaching	• Valuable teaching opportunity
• Limited opportunity for teaching on the ward	• Role modelling
• Poor quality of documentation	• Focus on discharge planning
• Missed opportunities	• Emphasis on the discharge plan within handover
	• Daily discharge updates
	• Effective communication with relatives and patients

Case studies

Communication with other healthcare and social care agencies

The single assessment process (SAP) was introduced as part of the 'National Service Framework for Older People' (DoH 2001). The SAP is a systematic, thorough assessment of need that is intended to prevent duplication of assessments across a range of different healthcare and social care agencies that may be involved in the patient's care.

Despite a specific project being established within the elderly care directorate in Birmingham, to focus on the introduction of the SAP, its implementation has been fraught with difficulties. Some of these problems can be directly attributed to the time it takes to complete the SAP within a busy acute hospital setting. Other problems appear to be associated with poor inter-professional and inter-agency communication processes. These are perhaps best illustrated by a recent example, where a patient admitted to an orthopaedic rehabilitation ward had brought with him seven completed SAP documents! The nurses involved in the SAP do seem to appreciate its importance, but a great deal more work still needs to be done in order to realise its full benefits for the patient and improve the process of communication with all involved.

Managing medication

Managing medication

The vast majority of patients who are discharged from hospital will be sent home with discharge medication. This may involve the patient adjusting their lifestyle to include a totally new medication regime or familiarising themselves with a newly adjusted medication regime. In either case, the changes must be carefully built into the discharge plan. A significant proportion of patients appear at clinics or other services with medication compliance issues. For example, in one extreme case a patient had simply stopped taking his medication because he was not advised that, when the medication supplied was nearing its end, he should order more. He did not realise that the medication was supposed to form part of his everyday life following discharge home.

It is vital for the ward pharmacist to ensure that patients and their carers are prepared for the management of medication following discharge. In addition, it is very helpful to involve the community pharmacist with the dispensing, delivery and follow-up

Simple discharge illustrated

(DoH 2005). Their knowledge and expertise should always be utilised as part of the discharge plan, however simple the discharge.

Tablets to take out

Tablets to take out

Completion of 'tablets to take out' requests (TTOs) is usually a fragmented process that is entirely dependent upon the practice standard set by the consultant team. At present, pharmacists are not routinely engaged in post-take ward rounds, where they could relieve junior doctors and provide a consistent high quality of service to patients. In areas where pharmacists have been employed they have been actively engaged in the transcribing of medications, and medication reviews to prevent unnecessary prescriptions (in cases where drugs remain unchanged, or where patients can be best advised to purchase over-the-counter medications).

All too frequently, a patient's discharge has been delayed overnight because of the late ordering and thus delayed arrival of TTOs. In extreme cases, this has resulted in transport arriving to collect a patient and being sent away! This is within the nurse's capability and remit, and could be easily rectified through better organisation and teamwork. The senior ward staff should have a central role in influencing how TTOs are to be prescribed. More importantly, they should be prescribed at the right time to effect good discharge practice.

Case study

Case study: Mrs S.

This example demonstrates how failure to plan simple discharge systematically can prolong a hospital stay.

Mrs S. is 78 years old and was admitted with a chest infection. She required a course of intravenous antibiotics and was proclaimed 'fit for discharge' five days after admission. Mrs S. lived alone in sheltered housing and she had no family. The warden was confirmed as the next of kin in the medical records. Mrs S. was fully independent and required no care package on discharge, constituting a simple discharge.

A nurse accompanied the medical team on the ward round, so it was acknowledged by the nursing staff that Mrs

S. could be discharged immediately. The ward round concluded at 9.40a.m. Mrs S.'s tablets to take home were not prescribed by the medical team until 1.55 p.m. and were not received in pharmacy for a further hour. A hospital car was booked to take Mrs S. home at 5 p.m. The car arrived on the ward to take Mrs S. home but was sent away as the tablets had not yet been received on the ward.

Pharmacy was contacted and the pharmacist explained that the tablets had been dispensed but were in transit with the porter. Portering was contacted and the nursing staff were assured that the tablets would be on the ward within the next 30 minutes. Nursing staff rebooked the hospital car for 6.30 p.m.

Mrs S. left the ward with take-home tablets and belongings and arrived back at her home just after 7p.m. On arrival, Mrs S. had a set of keys but not a front door key. The warden's office was closed, as she was only on site between 9 a.m. and 5 p.m. As it was getting late, the driver decided to take Mrs S. back to the accident and emergency (A&E) department. The time was 8.15 p.m. On arrival, Mrs S. was visibly upset and insisted that she wanted to go home and not remain in hospital for another night.

A&E staff contacted the warden, who confirmed that she would pick Mrs S. up and settle her into her home. Mrs S. arrived back home at 10.30 p.m. On investigation and reflection with the nursing team, two fundamental steps were found to have been omitted:

1. Not contacting the next of kin who in this case was the warden. The warden would have informed the nursing staff that the front door key was in her possession and would have ensured that she was available to welcome Mrs S. home.

2. Not prescribing the take-home tablets in a timely manner, on the ward round. On review of the prescription sheet, the intravenous antibiotics were discontinued and a seven-day course of oral antibiotics was prescribed. As no other medication was required, take-home tablets could have been prescribed prior to the day of discharge – if the medical and nursing teams had been thinking ahead.

If a discharge checklist had been in place, both the above points would have been highlighted 40 hours before discharge.

Tips for good practice:

- Hold weekly multidisciplinary team meetings
- Ensure good communications at nursing handover, focusing on discharge practice
- Involve the patients, in order to correctly identify and act upon their concerns
- Nurses should demonstrate leadership
- Don't assume knowledge and skills, and ensure that training on the job is part of the nurse's role
- Use the systems and tools that are already in place such as discharge checklists

References

Department of Health (2001). 'National Service Framework for Older People'. London: The Stationery Office.

Department of Health (2004). 'Achieving timely "simple" discharge from hospital: A toolkit for the multidisciplinary team'. London: The Stationery Office.

Department of Health (2005). 'Supporting people with long-term conditions: liberating the talents of nursing, caring for people with long-term conditions'. London: The Stationery Office.

Chapter 15

Refusing discharge or transfer of care

Siân Wade

Background

Hospitals across the UK have experienced problems when patients (or relatives on behalf of patients) have refused to go home or transfer to another setting. They may find different ways of delaying or preventing discharge, such as changing their mind about a care home once a place becomes available. Resolving delayed transfer of care is a national and local priority. From a legal perspective, once a person has been assessed as fit for discharge or transfer it could be argued that they are trespassing. There is no right to medical treatment.

Article 8 of the European Convention on Human Rights requires that each individual's rights and those of their family are respected. An individual may allege that transfer of care violates their rights under Article 8. However, consideration needs to be given to another person's equivalent Article 8 rights – to a bed in this case. A public authority can justify its decision to transfer a patient as a pressing social need, under the exception in Article 8 (2) for the protection of the rights of freedom of others. However, it would be a breach of Article 2, the right to life, if a patient who no longer requires medical treatment refuses to be transferred. This would deprive another patient of medical treatment, which could adversely affect that patient's condition and prognosis (DoH 2003).

Patients can use complaints procedures to delay discharge and this can eventually lead to a judicial review. It is therefore imperative that Trusts and staff are very clear and explicit with patients and families about what they can reasonably expect from their stay in hospital. If patients and their relatives are given appropriate verbal and written information throughout their contact with health professions, then their expectations should be realistic and reasonable. If, through the 'Direction on Choice' (LAC (92) 27 and LAC (93) 18), which recognises the importance of *patient choice*, a place is not available in the desired care home, alternative accommodation should be offered and means tested. If a patient is eligible for social services funding and refuses the transfer of care option, they effectively adopt the status of a self-funder and become responsible for making their own arrangements. If the patient is a self-funder, efforts should be made to assist them in finding alternative accommodation.

Resolution of such issues requires stakeholders across healthcare and social care agencies to collaborate closely. Most Trusts now have agreed inter-agency standards and policies to address these issues satisfactorily – although the process does take time (OHA/OSS 2002). For practitioners, it is vital to keep patients and their family members informed, to record all discussions, and to be clear about planned dates of discharge. In some settings, on admission patients receive a notice informing them of the expectations they can have of their stay. Where there is any suspicion of impending problems these need to be highlighted and referred to a higher level so that appropriate action can be instigated when appropriate.

Information exchange

Since all individuals are liable to forget things, especially those under some stress, it seems sensible to provide patients (and carers) with an information booklet detailing the plans for arrangements when they get home. Written information on any follow-up arrangements, and any patient education material, such as exercises or pressure relief, also need to be given (Johnson 2003). Where written information may be problematic, e.g. for patients who have difficulty reading, the use of tapes could be an option.

It is also important to assess, before discharge, the individual's understanding and ability to remember to take their medication. If problems are likely to be encountered, arrangements need to be made either for pre-dispensed tablets to be available, or for someone to remind them. Jim's case (see below) illustrates the importance of ensuring that discussions occur with any agencies or community staff who already know and care for the person. These discussions will shed light on any difficulties or problems with the proposed plans. Likewise, if any services are to be newly involved it is important to ensure that they are familiar with the plans and are happy with them.

Case study

Case study: Jim

Jim was an affable but rather cantankerous chap. At home he had a fluctuating venous leg ulcer related to his heart failure and obesity. Jim had a carer once a day, as this was all he would pay for, to help attend to his personal care and shopping, which he neglected badly. He seemed unable to remember to take his tablets. The district nurse had therefore arranged with the doctor for him to have daily diuretics in a dosset box, so that the carer could remind him to take them. Whilst not ideal, it was an adequate arrangement, when he did not refuse them or throw them on the floor.

Following discharge from hospital on one occasion, the district nurse arrived to attend to Jim's leg ulcers (which now only needed weekly compression) to find that Jim had been started on four times a day medication. However, the medication had been dispensed in boxes for him to take from. Hence they had sat unopened for five days after he had returned home. The district nurse had been in touch with the ward but this had not been discussed. She had to reorganise his medication, and has learnt to make sure that this issue is addressed should Jim be admitted again.

Finalising discharge arrangements

Finalising discharge

Most settings and services have a checklist that is completed as discharge arrangements are made. The list usually includes the date the arrangements are made and by whom, as well as a final checklist for the day of discharge. For the kind of patient under discussion here, significant areas that need to be addressed include:

- The availability of the house key if no one will be there to welcome them

- The availability of suitable clothing to go home in
- Clarity about transport and how this has been booked to tie in with care arrangements once home, if these are required

With the current challenges involving transport from hospitals, there needs to be a firm agreement that these patients will not be sent home late if there is a chance they will arrive after the carer has been asked to visit. Most team members are familiar with these requirements, but it is still vital to complete the checklists. They act as a form of communication, and also provide a means of auditing or checking back if problems do arise.

The consequences of delayed, failed or poor discharge

Delayed, failed or poor discharge

The consequences of delays or failure in transfer/discharge at different stages may be significant. There may be many different reasons for these problems (see below).

Possible reasons for failed transfer/discharge

- Failure to adequately assess and gain a realistic concept of required aftercare/on-going needs
- Failure to prepare for new/home setting, e.g. to recognise that care needs met in hospital cannot be met at home, such as need for equipment, help, advice, financial aids/benefits, access, preventative measures
- Failure to provide adequate or appropriate information about expected or potential pathway of care, settings involved and legal position
- Failure to keep the patient at the centre of the planning
- Failure to give adequate warning of date of discharge to carers or home
- Inability to provide services required
- Carers not turning up due to failures in communication
- Failure to provide adequate support, e.g. respite care/sitting, day/night care, counselling/emotional support

Many of these items may have been arranged or undertaken but communication has either failed or been inadequate.

Refusing discharge or transfer of care

If there is a breakdown in care once the individual has left the ward/service, the results can be even more devastating (see below).

Consequences of poor/failed care at home

- Distress to patients and carers – and loss of confidence/competence, possibly leading to regression
- Triggering of re-admission – to same or different hospital, causing discontinuity of care, which may be unnecessary
- Disruption of community services, loss of trust/respect
- Inability/failure to provide necessary care if not adequately planned
- Increased risk of iatrogenic disease, where the risk of hospital-acquired infection, further illness or greater disability increases due to being in hospital, particularly associated with a lengthy stay in hospital due to delay
- May increase pressure on beds

N.B. There will always be some discharges that are expected/predicted to fail where the discharge has in effect been:

- A trial discharge
- A self-proof discharge

References

Department of Health (2003). 'Discharge from hospital: pathway, process and practice'. London: The Stationery Office. (www.doh.gov.uk/jointuni)

Johnson A., Sandford, J. & Tyndall, J. (2003). 'Written and verbal information versus information only for patients being discharged from acute hospital settings to home'. Cochrane Review, in *The Cochrane Library 4*. Chichester: John Wiley and Sons.

Chapter 16

Case managers, advanced nurse practitioners and their interface with acute hospital services

Liz Lees and Barbara Mason

Background

Case manager and advanced nurse practitioner are two relatively new roles introduced into primary care trusts to enhance the District Nurse skills, while caring for patients at home with complex, long-term and possible exacerbations of acute conditions. Case Managers are responsible for the overall management of patients alongside the primary care team (including GPs as key players).

At the same time, systems to alert emergency care services have been established to identify patients with repeated admissions (regarded as the more vulnerable patients) within a specified time frame, e.g. within a month. Hence, the advanced nurse practitioners may institute care required in the community for groups of vulnerable patients, perhaps identified through repeated presentations at accident and emergency departments for treatment or through hospital admissions.

When the role has been fully established, case managers will probably work collaboratively with consultant nurses, emergency nurse and advanced nurse practitioners, discharge and intermediate care coordinators, and social care professionals (based within emergency care at a hospital or primary care trust) to make decisions regarding patients whose admission can be avoided and who could be managed at home. Thus, facilitating chronic care management and discharge pathways for patients will no longer necessarily be regarded as the domain of one organisation or group of staff. Instead, the responsibility will be shared across a spectrum of care services and relevant staff.

Case studies

In some instances, the case manager role is being introduced within a nursing framework, which also facilitates nursing practice at an advanced level, known as advanced nurse practitioners (ANPs). The approach is predominantly collaborative, utilising the skills of a whole team, supported by the continuity of care delivered by key players.

In the vast majority of cases, ANPs will be able to prescribe, and make referrals to all services, including requesting domiciliary visits and outpatient appointments. The key difference between case managers and ANPs is that Masters-level educational preparation is a prerequisite for all ANPs. These two new roles have been implemented to avoid inappropriate admission and re-admission to hospital. However, the opposite situation may also occur, in which a case manager or ANP may appropriately request a re-admission to hospital. These roles are supported by a Royal College of Nursing competency framework launched for the care of people with long-term conditions in August 2005 (DoH 2005).

Finally and importantly, case managers and ANPs are not the only new roles to be introduced to reduce re-admissions and improve the patient discharge experience. Actively managing patients and supporting self-care is at the heart of government policy development. One example of the new systems and processes that the NHS is seeking to learn from is Kaiser Permanente (KP), an integrated healthcare organisation based in California, in the USA. With KP it is likely there will be new information technology systems to promote and guide the appropriate access of different 'levels of health assessment' within Emergency Areas.

What are the benefits of having case managers?

Case managers

- They can improve communication between the primary and secondary care interface
- They can improve the process of discharge planning, by allocating responsibility to a key named person in the patient's discharge plan
- They can improve the quality of patients' care by facilitating a greater continuity of care from the nurses directly looking after them

- They can promote patient/carer/family involvement in discharge planning
- They may reduce admissions and decrease healthcare costs (Naylor *et al.* 1999)
- They offer a positive way to improve discharge planning knowledge among emergency care staff

Case study

Case study: M.

An 82-year-old lady, M., with moderate dementia and chronic obstructive pulmonary disease (COPD), had been in hospital for a month due to exacerbation of her COPD. She had been discharged and had been at home for two days. The district nurses had been asked to go in and dress her sacral pressure sore. During their visit, they became concerned about her condition and asked the community matron/assertive case manager (CM) to visit to review her condition. As the CM was still in training, she asked me to accompany her.

When we arrived at the house, M. was sitting in the chair looking very pale and grunting. M. was being looked after by her sister B. B. was distressed because M. had returned from hospital with marked mental deterioration. It was immediately obvious that M. was acutely ill. On examination it was found that M. had a raised temperature (pyrexial) with low oxygen saturation, and had an acute chest infection. I discussed with B. how ill her sister was and whether she wanted me to send her back to hospital. B. was adamant that her sister would not want to go back to hospital even though she knew there was a possibility that her sister might die.

I decided to put all measures together. I tried to phone the GP to let him know the joint decision made but it was the surgery's half day. I prescribed salbutamol nebules and oxygen to bring immediate relief and an antibiotic for her chest infection. We phoned the local pharmacist who agreed to deliver the oxygen cylinders, nebules and antibiotics to the home. We went back to our base to get a nebuliser and oxygen tubing. The CM set this up and showed B. how to use the nebuliser and the oxygen cylinder.

The GP out-of-hours service was informed by fax that this lady was acutely ill but the relatives did not wish her to be sent to hospital. M. was washed and made comfortable in bed by the CM, and the district nurse evening service came to monitor her condition and make her comfortable for the night. My fellow advanced nurse practitioner, H., came that evening to relieve the CM. There was another discussion with B. and H. about the possible outcome of M.'s illness.

The next day I phoned the GP to discuss the previous day's events, and he was surprised at all we had done with M. I discussed starting oromorph at night to help settle M. and improve her breathing and we agreed that this would help. I visited the next day and there was a remarkable turnaround in M.'s condition. The district nursing team were undertaking oral care, pressure area care and baseline observations. The intermediate care rapid response team agreed to call twice a day, at lunchtime and in the evening. The continuing healthcare coordinator was also asked to visit, as it was believed that M. was in the palliative phase of her disease.

Today M. is going strong, as she recovered so well from this illness with all the support received at home.

Case study

Case study: S.

An 81-year-old lady, S., had interstitial lung disease, rheumatoid arthritis and coronary heart disease. (She had received a coronary bypass graft in 1994.) I was asked to see S. by her assertive case manager/community matron, as S. was acutely ill and adamant that she did not want to go back into hospital.

S. is cared for by her daughter who has given up her job to care for her. S. is a very independent person, who refuses to have a bed downstairs and insists on sleeping on the settee in the living room. This lady is pyrexial with purulent sputum, increased respirations, inspiratory crackles and dullness on percussion on the left and right bases. Her daughter L. is doing an excellent job of giving her regular fluids and small frequent meals and S. is already on a daily dose of 5mg prednisolone and an antibiotic for a urinary tract infection.

S. is very thin. Although the skin is unbroken on her

sacrum, the area is red and she has to be encouraged to move position regularly. S. looks well hydrated. She has no problems with her bowels and her urine revealed nothing abnormal (NAD). After examining S. I had a discussion with her and L., to make absolutely sure that they did not want an admission to hospital. They made it very clear that they were happy for S. to be treated at home.

I phoned the GP's surgery to get the blood results from blood taken by the GP two days before. I was pleased to find that all these results were normal and that S. had not been dehydrated or anaemic. I shared my findings with the GP, and told him that I would start S. on an antibiotic recommended for chest infection, and that I would send a sputum specimen. S.'s oxygen saturation was low, due to her illness. Oxygen was therefore ordered and delivered within the four-hour period requested.

S. received daily visits from me, and her daughter was offered support by our team social worker. He was able to arrange for a sitter service to give some respite, as L. was very tearful at times. S.'s sputum specimen came back showing a bacteria infection that was sensitive to the antibiotic therapy I had already started her on. S. has made a slow but good recovery. As an advanced nurse practitioner, I discussed with her and her daughter the long-term prognosis for her condition, and the fact that she will be susceptible to other chest infections. I emphasised the importance of picking up these infections and starting treatment early. I also kept the GP informed of changes in her condition and any drugs prescribed, so that he could update his records.

Case studies

References

Department of Health, NHS Modernisation Agency, Skills for Health (2005). 'Case management framework launched for the care of people with long-term conditions'. London: The Stationery Office.

Lees, L. (2005). 'A framework to promote the holistic assessment of older people in emergency care'. *Journal of Older People's Nursing*, 16 (10), 16–21. (www.nursingolderpeople.co.uk)

Naylor, M.D., Brooten, D., Cambell, R., Jacobsen B.S., Mezey M.D., Pauly M.V. & Sanford Schwartz, J. (1999). 'Comprehensive discharge planning and home follow up of hospitalised elders: a randomised controlled trial'. *Journal of the American Medical Association*, 281, 613–620.

Index

Index